CARING FOR THE CARER

CARING FOR THE CARER

Authored by

Zamena Hassan

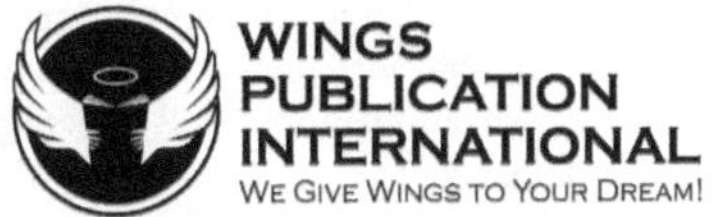

Disclaimer

This book has been published with all reasonable efforts taken to make the material error-free after the consent of the author. This book is sold subject to the condition that it shall not, by way of trade or otherwise, be lent, resold, or otherwise circulated without the copyright owner's prior written consent in any form of binding or cover other than that in which it is published and without a similar condition including this condition being imposed on the subsequent purchaser and without limiting the rights under copyright reserved above, no part of this publication maybe reproduced, stored in or introduced into a retrieval system or transmitted in any form or by any other means without the permission of the copyright owner.

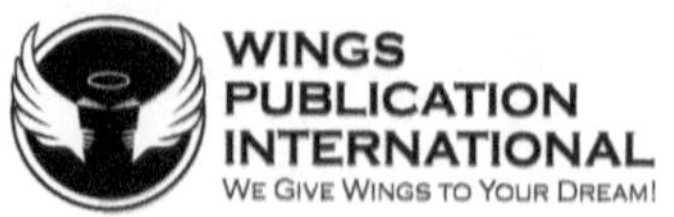

Registered Office- 907-Sneh Nagar, Sapna Sangeeta Road,
Agrasen Square, Indore – 452001 (M.P.), India
Website: http://www.wingspublication.com
Email: mybook@wingspublication.com

First Published by WINGS PUBLICATION 2024
Copyright **Zamena Hassan** 2024

Title: **CARING FOR THE CARER**
Price: AED 55 | $19 | PKR 999
All Rights Reserved.
ISBN 978-93-6006-797-7

LIMITS OF LIABILITY/DISCLAIMER OF WARRANTY

Dedication

I dedicate this book and my life to my father and mother, love you mummy and papa.

Acknowledgements

I am most grateful to God for giving me this beautiful life and everything around me.

I would like to thank my mentor and guide, Dr. Kailash Pinjani, for holding my hand metaphorically, through my entire journey of book-writing. I would never have done it without your support and guidance. Thank you.

I would like to thank my brothers, sisters, nephews, nieces, all the spouses and the rest of my immediate family for being supportive and patient with me while writing this book. Thank you for being part of my whole life's journey. Love you guys!

I would like to thank Farah R., Zahra and Ali H, Javeed P, Sheroz K, Youlla, Sawsan, Atul E., Dariusz G., and many others for being my constant support and confidantes. Love all of you!

I would like to thank all the doctors, (especially Dr. Lei Zheng, Dr. Richard Tuli, and Dr. Maroun El Khoury) and nurses who took care of my parents with such love and patience. I could not have made it through without you all. (Johns Hopkins Hospital, Cedars-Sinai Hospital, Adventist Hospital, American Hospital in Dubai)

I would like to thank everyone who crossed my path in this life journey of mine. Thank you very much.

Preface

When my mom became sick in Toronto, Canada, we took her to Hong Kong, China, for treatment. Then we moved to the United States of America (USA) for better treatment: first to Johns Hopkins Hospital in Baltimore, then to Cedars-Sinai Hospital in Los Angeles. Eventually, we brought her back to Dubai, the United Arab Emirates (UAE), where she lived for another year and passed away. Both my parents received treatments in Belgium, the USA, Pakistan and the UAE throughout their lives. My parents, two of my siblings and I were born in the Congo. I had two surgeries there and one surgery in Pakistan. I have assisted my parents and siblings with most of their procedures and treatments throughout the world. So, it suffices to say that all these experiences combined provide me with a thorough understanding of the kinds of hospitals and treatments found around the world.

When I was caring for my mother, I felt really isolated and lost. I kept looking for some guidance as a carer and found myself alone with no one to reach out to. In Los Angeles, there were support groups, but none were within a feasible distance. Inevitably, whenever I left my mom for too long or went far, she would get a fever or something, and I would have to rush back. I learned early on that I couldn't go very far while I was caring for her. My mom was the only one who semi-understood what I was going through, as she was always helping people in the family and the community and had seen others go through the carer's journey. There were a few who appreciated what I was doing. One person even commented: "You are like a robot, how do you do so much non-stop in a day?" Someone joked with my mom, who had a huge heart and helped everyone: "Noorjahan, even you couldn't do as much as Zamena is doing." Many were quick to judge me and my actions. Meanwhile, they never once asked what I was going through or how I was feeling. To be fair, no one knew what to do or feel, as everyone was going through his or her own emotional roller coaster. I think generally people don't know what to say or do in these situations. It's not anybody's fault really. We were never given a manual on how to behave in such circumstances unfortunately.

One of the doctors I became close to was complaining that he had had a long day and was too busy for me. I told him jokingly, "You are complaining when you work only 12 hours a day. I am on call, working 24/7. I don't even get a day off, so please don't try to get pity from me!" He agreed. The same doctor had told me: "If you want to take care of others, you have to first take care of yourself. You are no good to others if you aren't good to yourself." Taking care of myself? I didn't even understand what that meant. I was always taught: Take care of others, and God will take care of you. Don't be selfish. Don't put yourself before others. What was this man talking about?

Today, I am able to understand what he was saying. He meant - be kind to yourself. Take care of yourself in a 'good', kind of, selfish way, more like in a way of self-care. Self-care is good. It makes you happy and healthy in order to do more good. There is no point in pushing yourself to limits beyond what you can bear, only to fall apart after and lose yourself in the process. Putting the pieces back is hell. It leaves you unable to take care of yourself, and you get fed up with doing things for others. It is not healthy, neither physically, emotionally or mentally. Moreso, it makes you forget about yourself so much that you lose out on your own life and you don't even realize what is happening. You wake up one day ten years older with nothing to show for it. This book is about my experience of taking care of my parents and what I felt when I woke up one day too late to realize - wow, what just happened?

My parents both got diagnosed with blocked arteries on my 40th birthday in Hong Kong. We had gone there to get my dad checked by the cardiologist. Both my parents got their check-ups and needed stents put in their hearts. That was 2012, December 4. My mom was diagnosed with cancer in June 2013. She passed away 2016 January 1. My brother-in-law was diagnosed with lung cancer in December 2016 (again around my birthday). My dad passed away on March 18, 2021. My brother-in-law passed away in 2022 on July 6. His mom, who was extremely close to me, passed away 2 weeks later. Forward a few months later, it was now 2022, December 4, my 50th birthday…this is when I woke up to my new reality. Everything had changed.

Ten years is a long time. Ten years is the difference between your body being flexible and agile and getting body aches and stiffness. Ten years is the difference between being someone who can eat anything you want and being healthy without thinking, to now needing all kinds of medicines for diabetes, blood pressure, cholesterol, acid reflux, etc. Ten years is a decade, a lifetime. Ten years is how many new iPhones? How many soccer World Cups? Cricket World Cups? How much has technology changed in 10 years? How many wars took place in ten years? How many epidemics in ten years? How many fashion and music trends change in a decade? The world changed while I was oblivious, and most importantly, I changed. My heart stayed young, but when I looked in the mirror, it was someone I didn't recognize. My body didn't look familiar, nor did it move in the same way. Diabetes messed with my nail beds, and stubborn belly fat intensified with menopause kicking in. I was stuck in a 50-year-old body but thought still like the 40-year-old who felt 30. Inevitably, I ended up hanging out with 30-35-year-olds as they are single people now taking interesting courses and doing fun things. Thank God I had my 40s and 50s friends from before, haha, but they are all married with kids and not very spontaneous. (Sorry guys!)

This forced me to reassess my life. I now had no one to answer to other than God. I had no one in my life that I loved to come in the way of my relationship with Him either. My faith was super strong, but I realized that I was very alone and had no career or family of my own therefore, no structure in my life. It wasn't a very nice place to be. I thought about the years that had gone by and wondered if I could have done things differently. I thought of all that I had learned, could I use it for something bigger than myself? What if I could help people in a way that they could still be carers to their loved ones but would not have to deal with the aftermath that I ended up with? How could I help them dodge the bullets I had somehow managed to get hit with?

Don't get me wrong. I don't regret a single day of my time with my parents, and I would do it all over again if I had to. But my parents never had to take care of their parents for so long, or at all. So this was all new for everyone, not just me. I wish I had someone there to guide me and my family on how to do this right so no one had to lose out on elements of their life before their time. This journey has been a beautiful blessing, but the hiccups might not have been necessary. All these things pushed me to put my experiences and feelings out in the world. When I didn't know how to begin, Facebook brought me Dr. Kailash Pinjani's ad: "Writing for Success in 30 Days." I had always wanted to write but didn't know how to structure my thoughts on paper. The writing part was easy. Ask the people on my Facebook and Instagram pages, they have to bear with my writing all the time. I can write for hours and forever. But writing for a worldwide audience was daunting, and I didn't feel confident enough to put my words out there without a guide. I found my mentor in the being of Dr Kailash. I had always wanted to write fiction based on reality, but his workshop convinced me otherwise. Non-fiction was not my kind of literature, nor was baring my soul an option, But, fortunately or unfortunately, here I am today writing about my most intimate experiences for anyone who will read it because the only thing I know for sure about myself, in this life, is that I want to help as many people as I can in whatever way I possibly can. So, for better or for worse, this is here to stay as my legacy. Thank you for reading it, and may it help your life in whatever little way it can. If nothing else, it can be used to support a plate or an uneven table leg. At most, may it provide you with solace and companionship in this lonely and spiritually beautiful journey. I pray your loved one has a swift and full of ease recovery. May you have all their blessings, and take care of yourself.

This book is my labour of love to the world to help any family out there in their time of difficulty. It is my gift to the single female carers from the subcontinent who are giving up their lives to take care of their parents while forgetting about their own needs and wants of life. If any of my experiences can help preserve a new caregiver's health - mental, physical and emotional, then this attempt of mine will have been worth the effort. Sharing my caregiver's life with you all will hopefully give you a heads-up on what to expect and what to be prepared for. My wish is that it serves as a map, a companion and a starting point on your journey as a caregiver. Most importantly, I hope this book helps you prevent the mistakes I made when taking care of my parents.

The book's name is 'Caring for the Carer', but my experience is primarily as a daughter taking care of her mother and later for her father. Therefore, the content is more of "Carer to Parents", and it does not include anything about a person caring for a sick spouse or an ill child, for that matter, any other close relation like a sibling, etc. That kind of care probably has a completely different set of emotions and tasks, which I have not mentioned. Some of the experiences I have been told about (and maybe one day I can write some sequels from other people's experiences) are:

- I've seen my mother work like a superwoman for about a year and a half, taking care of my cancer-stricken father till he passed away. However, he was somewhat selective in who took care of him. For some tasks, he was okay with his brothers performing and not my mother, whereas he didn't want his younger sister to help him at all.

- I see my neighbour taking care of his cancer-stricken wife and juggling his life, managing his daughters' schooling and homework, etc., along with his office work and his wife's chemo sessions & surgeries.

- My classmate from college, a stubbornly jovial and impractical chap, went through a 13-hour surgery to remove most of his gastrointestinal system and drove himself home a week after getting discharged from the hospital.

There are many such cases which I could not include in this

little guidebook. I hope one day to be able to address all these other aspects as well.

In the meantime, I would like to make you aware of certain issues I faced after my time as a carer. Namely, assimilating back into society after going through all these events was super challenging. Again, finding people to relate to is important, but it is a difficult task in itself. Just like you, everyone else who has been through the same type of events will be just as scared and weirded out as you and will hesitate to speak about it. So, be vocal and proactive. Don't be shy to speak.

The social aspect I found the hardest to deal with because I had been living in hospitals and dealing with death and dying issues for years on end. I couldn't relate to anyone anymore, I felt like I was from a different planet. They talked about petty and useless things; regular life looked very mundane to me. When people around me talked about acquiring material things, I just found them very petty and frivolous. Maybe I became judgmental and, in a way, a bit egotistical in thinking that I am better than everyone because I had dealt with the 'real' hard stuff that life is all about. This was a big mistake on my part, and I realized it much later. This experience should make you more humble and grateful, not egotistical.

The fact that you are chosen to be of service to others, especially your parents, the people who brought you into this world and took care of you when you were not able to take care of yourself, is a huge blessing in your life. It is an opportunity, when taken and done right, to provide you with so much peace while doing it and afterwards. Your parents' appreciation and blessings will propel you in such wonderful directions that you have to wait and watch later. Even if they seem angry and picky, they will still appreciate you being there for them. If not, then the Universe is always there to reflect your goodness back to you in ways unimaginable.

Index

CHAPTER 1

FINDING OUT PARENT IS SICK WITH CHRONIC OR TERMINAL ILLNESS

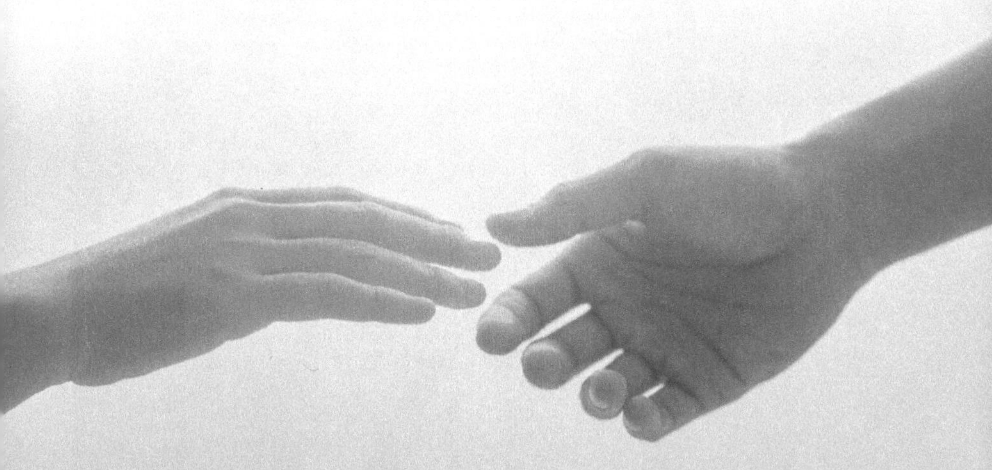

Reaction

You are not alone! For all of us who are lucky to have our parents with us till a late age, it is inevitable that they will get some illness or the other, except for the lucky few who will die of old age symptoms. This book will focus on parents who will get cancer or other terminal illnesses which require one or more of their adult children to look after them with the same care and concern as the parents did for their kids when they were young. (Rabbir hum huma kama rabbayani sagheera - "My Lord, have mercy upon them as they brought me up [when I was] small." Quran - Surah Al-Isra, 17-24) The one who spends the most time and is the most responsible for the parent's health and well-being is the main caregiver or carer. Definition of Caregiver or Carer: "A caregiver gives care, generally in the home environment, for an ageing parent, spouse, another relative, or unrelated person, or for an ill, or disabled person without payment." (www.hopkinsmedicine.org/health/caregiving/being-a-caregiver)

When we first find out our loved one has a terminal illness, our brains and body freeze. We get paralyzed with fear and anxiety. Most people have never had to deal with doctors, hospitals, or anything medical in their lives before this point. We are, for the most part, not exposed to people who are sick or dying as we grow up. Therefore, it has never been important to understand the simple CBC tests, nor has one had to deal with gadgets like glucose and blood pressure monitors. Basic care with thermometers and crutches for broken bones is probably the most we have had to deal with. Well, guess what? This new situation will require us to get into gear and start learning new vocabulary like 'orthostatic' blood pressure and understanding the difference between x-rays, MRIs, CT scans, PET scans, ultrasounds, and myriad other names of procedures, surgeries and treatments. Get ready for an 'information overload'. Normally, one should be well prepared! Unfortunately, at this moment, one is not bestowed with the privilege of time. You have to learn on the job; literally, you are to be thrown into the deep end of the water, not knowing how to swim with all this emotional turmoil going on inside. Getting the mind to work while the heart pounds with pain will be the biggest challenge at this time.

Due to our cultures, many of us do not like to make illnesses public knowledge. Please do let people know. It is extremely important to let family and friends know. Then only will others come forward and say, oh, so and so had the same illness, too. This will help you because, firstly, you will learn which hospital, doctor and treatments are viable options. Sharing experiences is great as you learn what to do and what not to do for your patient. Secondly, as more and more people find out, they will pray for the patient, and prayers have a power that is above and beyond any treatment the patient will get. We all need prayers, and, above all, we need God on our side. So reach out to family, friends, and your community, including places of prayer that you may be affiliated with. In fact, these are the people who will support and carry you through this journey- they are your backbone, your emotional and spiritual tribe.

My uncle was in the hospital once, bleeding internally. The hospital had the machines but didn't have a technician who knew how to use the machine. The doctor had just come from the USA. She told us: Pray, I can only fix this once the bleeding stops and prayers are the only hope for him to survive right now. We prayed for ten days, the bleeding stopped, and they managed to save him.

Responsible people and Responsibilities

The main carer will have to be a flexible, caring, patient, loving and forgiving person. Just like when you were a child, as you depended on your parents, your parents will now depend on you. Even though they have been used to making decisions and being in control of their lives, their confidence and decision-making powers will be blunted and affected by age and/or the illness.

The responsibilities of the carer will include:

1) Researching the disease

2) Choosing the hospital

3) Choosing the doctors

4) Choosing the treatment and way forward

5) Organizing the medications

6) Organizing food

7) Organizing exercise

8) Organizing alternate treatments

9) Organizing additional therapies

10) Transporting patients to appointments and attending appointments

11) Making important decisions with the patient

12) Staying overnight at the hospital or at home with the patient at times or all the time

13) Knowing the rights of the patient and fighting for them

14) Organizing assistive technologies if needed

15) Providing emotional support

16) Dealing with the insurance companies

17) Organizing the financial requirements

Time Factor Unknown

Cancer, strokes, paralysis, dementia, Alzheimer's, and other debilitating maladies do not come with expiry dates. The length of time the person will take to recover or not might be determined by a doctor, but no one can guarantee it, not even the doctor himself.

"Verily the knowledge of the Hour is with Allah (alone). It is He Who sends down rain, and He Who knows what is in the wombs. Nor does anyone know what it is that he will earn on the morrow: Nor does anyone know in what land he is to die. Verily with Allah is full knowledge and He is acquainted (with all things)." (Quran - Surah Luqman, 31:34)

I know a lady who was diagnosed with fourth-stage lung cancer and was given 6 months to live. She was told to wrap up her life because there was no way she would see Christmas that year. She saw about 25 Christmases after that.

Doctors are knowledgeable, but they are not God. They make mistakes, too, but they are definitely NOT omniscient. Do the treatments and everything possible, although, at the end of the day, one must trust God and submit to His will.

Even when a person goes into remission and recovers beautifully, the fear of the disease recurring remains. Every time you go for a scan, there is a scare, an uncertainty, that this time something will come up. The whole family is tense, not just the patient. As the primary carer, you will have to be prepared to go through it over and over again. When cancer comes back, it comes back way stronger. Life gets turned upside down again. You have to be ready for this, or maybe next time, you can hand the baton to a sibling.

You have to ask yourself some questions:

1) Can I afford to take time off from work indefinitely (again) financially?

2) Will my career be affected by gaps in my resume?

3) Can I afford to emotionally and mentally take on this responsibility?

4) Will my own spouse and children be able to handle me taking on this responsibility?

5) If I don't take this responsibility, will I regret it?

6) If there is no one else to do it, who will do it if I don't?

7) If I don't take care of my parents, will I expect my kids to take care of me?

8) How much care can be outsourced to nurses and other carers to keep the dignity of the ill parent intact?

9) What duties and obligations as a child of the ill parent are you prepared to follow, and which are you willing to forego?

10) How much can I do for my parents with love, and what are my limits?

11) When the care stops being loving and starts becoming forced, causing frustration and friction between you and the patient, stop! Take a step back and assess the situation again. This may be a time to think of your own well being by handing the responsibilities over to a sibling.

If you are single, there will be a lot of pressure on you to be the carer by default as you don't have obligations like having your own children or a spouse. This does not mean you 'have' to do it. You have a life, too, even though it may not be the life everyone expects you to have in our culture. Just because you didn't follow the scripted path of life doesn't mean your life is any less important than that of others.

Also, we have no idea how long this 'job' is for. Remember, you only have so many years to find that spouse and have your children. The ones who already have their own family unit could be the ones to take care of the parents. You need to focus on securing your life and settling down. Wouldn't it be lovely to have your parents at your wedding? Wouldn't it be amazing for your children to also see their grandparents get spoiled by them as only a grandparent does best? People in our culture never see it this way. They just fall to the easy justification of, oh, you are single and free, so you should do it. The married siblings say, "We are married and too busy, so we cannot give up our lives". But isn't the fact that they have emotional support from their spouses a good reason for them to have this emotional and mental stress? The single person doesn't get refuelled by anyone. Besides, the parent is not just the single person's parent solely, they are all the siblings' parents. Therefore, the responsibilities are everyone's equally, just as we demand equal attention from the parents, the parents deserve equal attention from each of their kids.

Another point to consider, which nobody does, is that married people are the ones the parents have been running around for the most. Parents are always making sure the married ones are happy in their marriages. Furthermore, they spend oodles of time babysitting the kids and so much more. It is only natural that the married ones return the favour and feel more vulnerable and empathetic towards the ill parent to give back what they have gotten. Most importantly, parents are forever saying: "When you become a parent, you will understand!" Furthermore, married people always love to say, "You single ones don't know the love between a child and parent because you don't have children." So how come now, when it's time to show that love, it's the single ones that come forth? To top it all off, children do what they see their parents do. If you don't look after your parents, chances are your children won't look after you. So, even if it is just for selfish reasons, look after your parents whether you are married or single.

Besides, the person who takes this responsibility doesn't have to be the sole person doing everything, although they do need to be the director of the whole situation. As the carer, you can delegate responsibilities to siblings, neighbours, helpers, etc, but you have to be the one to make sure no one slips. If someone gets sick or can't be there for the patient, a substitute has to be chosen, and usually, that will be you. It's a 24/7 job, and the length of treatment and care is unknown. One has to be mentally prepared to make a life-long decision (i.e. the patient's life or yours, in case you die while taking care of them). Yes, you can die, too, in the process. Death doesn't come with a warning, and we know very well that it has 'no requirements': any age, any day, any time is time - so technically, we are all dying since the time we are born!

Just because the illness has a feeling of impending doom

attached to it, that doesn't mean the patient is dead already. They are still here and still living, so let them live while they can. While my mom was sick, we thought oh my god, she has limited time on earth, so she has to be the highest of priorities, and the whole world needs to be secondary as she will go first. But imagine, a few months after her initial procedure, one of her doctors went to a yacht party where a cyclone hit, and he fell off the boat and drowned. God bless his soul. It was a big shock to our system. That was the day we realized that even my mom needed to keep up with people and continue regular social interactions to give people the time and attention they deserved in case they left this world before her. After that, so many people passed away, and in a weird way, it helped her and us to appreciate the time we had left here on earth.

Decision-making person

Illnesses require many different life-altering decisions. These decisions have to be made by the patient, their spouse, and the family as a whole. Even then, there has to be one spokesperson who will liaise with the doctors, etc, and usually, this role will be played by the main carer, who is you.

It is imperative that you take into consideration the patient's decision to do the treatment or not or which treatment they should do. It's their body, and they know best what they can handle or not. For example, you may feel objectively that they should take the chemotherapy that is more aggressive, but if they know their body cannot handle it, they may choose to take another chemotherapy or treatment that has fewer side effects. Some chemotherapy causes the patient to lose their hair, so if the person doesn't want that to happen, they may choose a less aggressive treatment with side effects they can handle. At the end of the day, it's their life, and they are responsible for their body and its well-being. You are just an enabler and support to make their life easier and comfortable.

You and the rest of the family will want the patient to fight hardest, so you will find it tough for the patient to skip or delay treatments, but you have to respect the patient's needs and wants. It is a very difficult situation to accept, especially when the possible consequences of such actions are on one's mind. What we must accept and believe is that whatever happens is the will of God, and we can only do our best and leave it up to Him. In Islam, this is called 'tawakkul'. In Christianity, we call it trusting God to do the best for you. Every religion and spirituality has a concept of doing your best and letting go of the outcome. The Higher Energy knows better than you what is best for you.

There are many situations where we can go and find the best treatments and best hospitals in the world if we have the means to do so, but in the end, the patient doesn't recover. Other times, I know that someone has gotten mouth cancer yet has refused allopathic treatment in a third-world country and chosen to go to their village to get treated. That person is still alive and healthy today, while the ones who travelled to the best nations and got the best treatments in the world have passed away. So the moral of the story seems to be: Do the best you can and give them the best they want, the rest is up to their fate and/or destiny.

At this point, one has to look deep into one's soul and trust the Universe submitting wholly. Why some people survive and why others don't is something no one understands to this day. Each person's tumour has a different makeup, even if the name of the cancer is the same. Moreover, each tumour in the body of the patient can have unique and varied characteristics under the umbrella of a common cancer diagnosis. The identical chemo or treatment may not work the same way on other cancer patients as similarly diagnosed patients. So why does one individual go into remission after getting treated in a village, but the other one may go to the best hospital in the world and yet they succumb to the disease's deadly target? After seeing over a dozen family members and friends go through their painful journeys of receiving cancer treatment through the years, with some surviving and others not, I do not see a logical pattern to the reasons for survival. Everyone can have their own theories, but I don't think even doctors can predict the outcomes. If one believes in spirituality, the only way to make sense of this phenomenon is to accept that God decides who is to live through and who not. Fate is the answer; we will die the day we are meant to and not one day less or more.

We all have a purpose in this life. Until we do not serve the purpose we have come to fulfil, we will remain in this world. I have seen some people forego all treatment yet have recovered through sheer will, changing only their nutrition, doing yoga and meditation. For allopathic and non-spiritual people, this is seen as madness. For them, foregoing allopathic treatment is almost akin to committing suicide. There is tremendous pressure on all of us to do chemo and radiation, take pills, do scans with radiation and so on. The doctors instil such fear in us that we dare not skip these allopathic treatments. We tend to add naturopathic, homoeopathic, and nutrition-based treatments to the allopathic treatments even though it has not been proven that eating and abstaining from foods helps calm inflammation and slow down the deterioration of cells.

There are many non-medical hospitals in India, China and other parts of the world. Many people have gotten cured without treatment: Anita Moorjani's "Dying to be Me" (cancer), Terry Wahl's

"The Wahls Protocol" (Multiple Sclerosis and other autoimmune disorders), Jill Bolte Taylor's "My Stroke of Insight" (Stroke) and Joe Dispenza have many examples of people who have recovered from illnesses - to name a few. Among the alternative treatments, the following are recommended for additional therapies use of Turmeric/Curcumin, Moringa Leaves, Black Seed oil, Magnesium, Vitamins, Juicing, walking, hydration, salt and coffee baths, meditation, bio-resonance therapy, frequency balancing, oxygen therapy, cottage cheese and flaxseed therapy (Budwig Diet), exercise, yoga. These, amongst others, are some ways people are trying to ward off or reverse these illnesses, even though medical research doesn't promote their usage.

At the end of the day, we all have to die. The only thing that is guaranteed in our lives if we are born is that we are going to die one day. It may sound morose and bleak, but that is the reality and the only truth we have to hold on to. Nothing between birth and death is guaranteed or promised. Yet, we base all our lives and hopes on the dreams we have about the in-between part. We focus on everything except for the fact that we are definitely going to die someday. Why is it that we are so scared of dying when that is all we are guaranteed? Why do we focus on everything else other than the most important step of our life, which we know is to come? Even the healthiest of people don't always make it to 100 years of age. The bottom line is that we can try our hardest to be safe and healthy, but a day will come when we have to leave this world and go on to whatever may come after. Who decides this for someone who does everything right with their food, exercise and life in general? Clearly, they can only control their ageing and lifespan to a certain extent, then there is a force above, a wisdom which decides: now your time here is over.

The soul that we have inside of us connects us to the rest of the people in this world, coming together as one uniting force: some refer to this as the Universe, Energy, God, Allah, Bhagwan, and so on. We all may refer to the same entity with different names. Regardless, this entity is the one that decides who goes and when that time is. When our purpose here on earth is fulfilled, the soul is then called back to reconnect to the divine Source. As a carer, we are literally helping the patient conclude their purposeful journey of this life while guiding them back to the Source. The job of a carer may be seen as very easy and simple, but it's an extremely intense and complicated one. We are carers and spiritual workers in one. We work in this world and carry the patient over to the next. We are the last people to make an impact on the soul of the body of the patient before it makes the journey back to reconnect with God. We are chosen for this job for a reason. The impact this will have on our lives is not something we know when we start doing it. The blessings one receives in doing this job are endless, and the fruits we reap are beyond imagination. We are literally plugging into the unending source of abundance directly as a sick/suffering person's prayers go straight to God as they balance delicately between this world and the next. It is almost like they have one leg in this world and one in the next. I truly believe this is the reason for the success and beautiful rewards a carer experiences with the blessings they receive from taking care of their loved ones on their journey to the next world. Some people may think it a myth, and it feels so much of a cliche when people say: you are doing such a great job, you will be rewarded for taking care of your parents. But I am a living example of this, and I am ever so grateful. I had no idea what would happen to me. I had no plan or direction. I went to a therapist and took care of my mental health. My personal trainer and nutrition guides have helped me get my physical body in shape. My doctors overlooked my need to put my health in order. My family and friends have helped me maintain my zest for life, which has enabled me to gain the confidence to get out there and join acting, film-making and all kinds of classes. My world has changed, and I am the happiest I have ever been.

It seems that whatever we run after in this life runs away from us. When we are desperate for something, it evades us. When we accept where we are and do our best to be the highest version of ourselves in a given situation, usually, the Universe starts sending all kinds of goodies to us. In the same way, when we accept our situation even in illness (which can be terribly hard), then submitting to God's will allows us to accept whatever decree He has in store for us. If we live, it's His will, and if we don't, it's His will, too. How can anything commanded by His will ever be bad? He knows best, and when we truly believe in that All-Merciful and All-Knowing and All-Caring God, then we can never doubt anything again. Strong faith and belief in His wisdom will allow us to gladly accept every decision of His. This is not to say that we shouldn't try or that we should just sit around waiting for His direction. No, always do your best. Get the best treatment possible, fight your hardest, be the most patient of humans, and have the most gratitude for each and every step along the way, but then leave the outcome to Him. Don't get attached to the outcome you want, allow Him to choose the best and then accept it graciously.

I used to tell my mom that when we pray to live longer, whether we are sick or not, won't God ask us what we are doing with the life he has already given us? Don't we need to show him what we would do with the life he extends for us? If we just keep saying, oh, if I have a longer time on this Earth, this is what I would do...if we don't do it now and show Him, then how is God supposed to trust that we will actually do it given an extension? Isn't it best to show Him now so that He believes it? And if our life gets cut off, then, hey, at least we started the ball rolling for someone else to continue!

Spouse's role: (depends on age)

A young spouse will be able to be the main carer for the person with the illness. As we grow older, our capacity to care for our other half gets limited. We have our own issues, and our hearts cannot bear seeing the most important person in our lives fight for their lives. In this case, we need the help of our children, although we still need to be an important part of the process. The carer, being the adult son or daughter, has to understand this need for the spouse to not feel useless or redundant. They are also getting older and need to feel cared for and respected in the process. If they are forgotten, they will age faster and will end up falling sick as well. To prevent this from happening, the carer has to remember to involve them in the decision-making process, and they should be involved in the 'caregiving' process to the best of their capabilities.

When my mother got sick, the first thing my uncle, whose wife had had lung cancer, told me was, "Make sure to take care of your dad." It was the best advice he could have given me. It is so easy to forget the spouse's well-being when the focus is on one parent. We have to remember that they have been each other's strength, and they have a relationship separate from just being your parents. It's only natural that the spouse will now try not to be mean and use their best behaviour toward the one going through the illness, and this will make them frustrated at times. Be patient with them and try to have compassion when they vent on you. They also need fuel for love as the ill spouse may not be able to give them the love they are used to getting. So try to give them as much love as you can, or else they will get weak, and then they might get sick too.

Remember, you saw your sick parent for parts of the days, months or years. The spouse shared a life 24/7 with this individual. They made decisions together and cared for you rather than asking you for anything. Now, the tables have turned for the first time, and no one knows how to handle or understand that yet. It is a learning curve for everyone involved. Be kind to and patient with each other, and that kindness will come back to you.

Second Opinion from other doctor/hospital

One of the ideas we grow up with in Southeast Asian, African and Middle Eastern cultures is that doctors are infallible. Doctors also tend to have the 'God' syndrome, whereby they think they know everything, and they usually don't like to listen to others. But we must remember that humans are fallible, even doctors, and most importantly, the patient's life is at stake here. So it is imperative that one gets a second opinion from another doctor, usually from another hospital, to make sure that the diagnosis, prognosis and treatment plans are all agreed upon. Nowadays, second opinions can be done online in different countries also. There is a fee involved in most cases for a second opinion. If one has the financial means, one can research the best doctor in the field of treatment to ask for their opinion on how they would proceed with the treatment.

Once treatment starts, it is very hard to undo any of the processes, and we do not want to regret any of the choices. Of course, sometimes we do not have the luxury of getting a second opinion due to either the lack of options or the restriction of time, i.e. in emergencies. Then, of course, one has no choice but to trust faith and go with whatever is available at the moment.

Another reason one should consider a second opinion is that there are always new treatments and options for surgery and other novel ways of treating the patient for the diagnosed illness. In my experience, from January to December of the same year, immunotherapy as a treatment for cancer went from the last line of treatment to the first line of treatment. Sometimes, if the doctor is older, they have lots of experience but may not be up to par with the new techniques and treatments. The younger doctors will have access to new treatments and will have new skills, but the lack of experience can serve as an impediment.

The hospital matters, too. Some hospitals can have great doctors but not the right equipment. Other hospitals can have all the latest equipment but the doctors do not have a good outcome in treating patients. One has to be extremely diligent in choosing the doctor and hospital balance to treat their loved ones. It is highly recommended to speak to others that have been through the same experience to get a better idea of the options available close to home.

Being home makes a huge difference in treating the individual. It gives the patient and the supporting family members a sense of familiarity and a sense of 'home' when the world is collapsing around them. Also, when the treatment is going on, it helps to be home to continue working and have a semblance of 'normality' to counteract the instability of the consequences of the disease. One of my mom's doctors gave us the best advice: "Do not make cancer your life." He meant to say the disease is a part of your life, not your whole life. Continue living your life with the treatment as an addition; continue focusing on yourself as a person. Do your treatment and get on as normally as you can.

How to be there for the patient when they find out

When the patient is first diagnosed with a chronic or terminal illness, the ground beneath seems to have blown open, and one is left unshielded by the storm coming on. It is an extremely shocking and scary feeling for the patient and family members, above all for the patient. In this instance, the patient will need a lot of support and physical care. It is a psychological and physical trauma effect which can only be balanced by lots of warmth, care and communication. Everyone will process the information differently, so there isn't just one answer. It is best to gauge the reactions and try to be there for each other as needed. Allowing for open discussions while sharing each one's fears and concerns will be a great way to make sure the family stays together.

If not handled carefully, the miscommunication or lack thereof can cause great rifts between members, resulting in colossal damage that may or may not be repairable for days, months, or years to come. This can lead to disunity in the family, causing regrets if conflicts are not resolved before the patient, God forbid, succumbs to the illness. These kinds of ruptures in families can lead to disharmony during the illness, which will lead to some parties not spending time with the patient because of other members. It can even lead to inheritance fights since one party may think the other didn't do enough to deserve anything, whereas the others did way more than them. In grief, the combination of wild emotions and regrets can be a deadly cocktail. People can be really mean at this time and may say things they don't mean. Hopefully, time will bring everyone together, and the venting everyone does before gets forgiven sincerely from all parties involved.

What choices do we have? Take treatment or alternative or nothing.

If the parent is elderly, sometimes the effect of the surgeries required, cancer treatments or other treatments/procedures may be too difficult to undergo for them. This may lead to the family and doctors choosing palliative care, which involves keeping the patient comfortable and pain-free with minimal treatment. This is a very difficult decision to take and even harder to accept since it highlights the fact that the patient will not ever recover. It takes away every ounce of hope.

If the patient is strong enough to go through surgeries and treatments, the doctors and patient, along with the family, will have to make some very difficult choices. These provide hope to the patient and the members of the family that the patient may recover. The ride may be bumpy and will require a lot of patience. Emotions will run wild and the journey is full of ups and downs but hope is what keeps us going.

Some people do not believe in medical treatments and may choose alternate treatments such as:

1) Homeopathic

2) Naturopathic

3) Hakim or tribal

4) Spiritual or religious treatment

5) Holistic or osteopathic treatment involves:

a) Yoga

b) Meditation

c) Food and nutrition

d) Psychological treatment

e) Faith related treatments

f) Chinese traditional medicine

Choosing to go without allopathic treatments can feel risky, but people have done it and have had amazing results. Other people do not believe in allopathic treatments like chemotherapy, as they may cause damage to extra organs along with trying to heal the tumour itself. Stem cell therapies and bone marrow transplants affect the whole body and can be life-threatening procedures, although the results are fantastic if successful. Brain tumours can require surgery on the brain, which can lead to epileptic seizures, paralysis and other complications. The Whipple's surgery leads to man-made diabetes, digestive issues and lower immunity since they remove the pancreas, bile duct, gallbladder and duodenum.

The above are just some examples of treatments related to cancer, which can be scary. Yes, these sound risky, but some people believe in allopathic treatments wholeheartedly and would not be able to handle skipping these options. Others have so much faith in homoeopathic and traditional medicine that they don't bother with allopathic treatments. There is a middle ground, though. Allopathic treatments aim at suppressing the disease. Homoeopathic treatments work with a holistic approach to cure the root cause and prevention of the disease. Most people these days choose to do allopathic treatment in parallel with homoeopathic treatment so that they complement each other. One should always ask the doctors to help you decide as the medicines can be counter-indicative and doctors will be able to guide you best.

CHAPTER 2

MEDICAL OBLIGATIONS

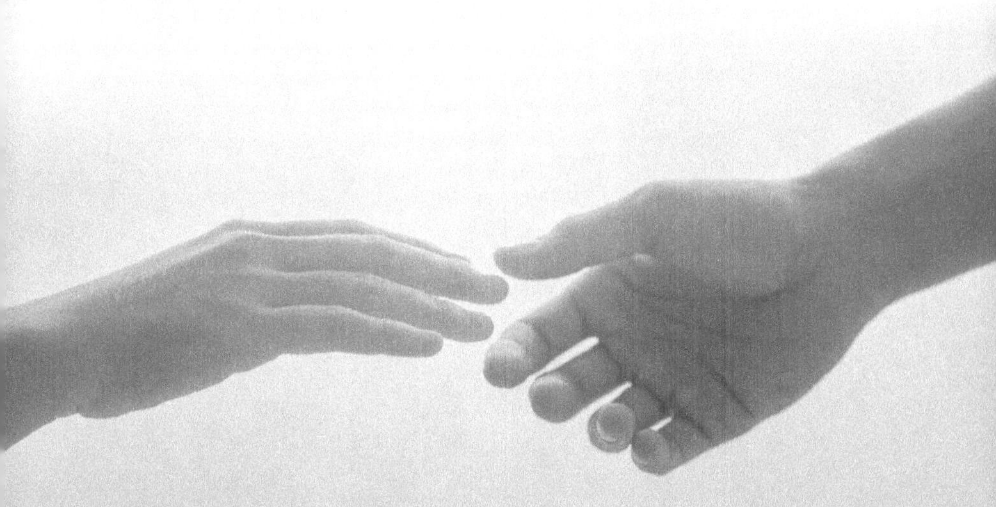

Researching the Disease

When a loved one gets diagnosed with a scary disease, it is a natural reaction to google the hell out of the disease. We are not doctors and hopefully we haven't had to deal with anything like it before. There are pros and cons to googling the disease as sites like WebMd are good but they give every scenario possible and may scare you more than necessary. These website doctors are not substitutes for real doctors and shouldn't be used to replace your doctor.

Also, they love to give you statistics on the prognosis of the disease. For example, they may say that there is a 10% chance of recovery or remission. Let's say there are 100 patients that they did the research on, which means that 10 out of a hundred went into remission. How does that help you? It doesn't because our natural tendency is to think, "Oh my god, 90 people didn't make it." The patient is not competing with other patients, nor is the patient helped by the other's recovery. The patient needs to focus on healing themselves and doing the best they can with all the treatments and nutrition in addition to keeping the mind positive and healthy. Moreso, they just have to focus on being the 11th person to recover, thereby becoming the positive statistic, if anything! Keeping their hopes high and working towards a positive outcome is the best way to fight the disease. As the carer, you will be around the patient the most. Therefore, you will be key in keeping this hope alive. The patient will tend to look towards you for encouragement and to boost their morale. Think of it as being a coach of a sports team. You cannot let them feel your stress or worries; otherwise, they will lose their focus and hope. When they lose hope, their body stops fighting, it's on you to pick them up and carry them through. You have to keep building their spirit and root them on always with a big smile and lots of love and positivity!

Choosing the Hospital (city/country/reputation)

If your country has good doctors and hospitals, then it's easy, stay home for treatment. That is definitely the best option always. But for the rest of us who do not have this luxury at home, we must get transported to another village, another town or city, or in some cases another country altogether.

Some of the things to be considered are:

1) Treatment for patient

2) Patient's ability to travel

3) Insurance coverage

4) Financial budget

5) Logistical concerns

6) Family support in the other location

7) Living arrangements in other locations

8) Visas if going to another country

Of course, the number one point of concern would be the

availability of treatment in the other location. Once that is pinpointed, then one has to see if the patient is able to travel, whether by car or flight. If that is possible and the patient has insurance coverage, one should see if the chosen hospital treatment is covered under the insurance coverage. Also, insurance is not the only concern for the financial budget. There will be other expenses, such as living arrangements, food, and travel to, from and within the new location.

Sadly, many people think insurance covers everything. In the States, Medicare kicks in when one is of retirement age, this ensures healthcare for the elderly. The free part of Medicare only covers hospitalization costs. The second part, which covers consultations, has to be paid for. The UK and Canada have NHS and OHIP, which provide free public healthcare for their residents. The UK has the option of private healthcare available at a cost, unlike Canada. Free public healthcare is a great concept since everyone gets the same care regardless of status and power, but then you have long waits for biopsies and surgeries, which can be life-threatening. In the UK, even if both options are available, the doctors work in both, so one would beg the question: why pay for something I can get for free? In countries like India, Pakistan and other third-world countries, the country does less for the people than the philanthropist families and religious groups. Private organizations have set up cancer hospitals, kidney care hospitals, hospices for end-of-life care, and so many other clinics, all for free or at a minimal cost.

My parents were of this calibre in a country where people don't have money to eat, and hospital care and free healthcare remain a lucid dream. They opened a 'Mother and Child' clinic in the remote part of Kinshasa, which provided women with pre-delivery, postdelivery and delivery of the child. These services were offered at a minimal cost of 5$ with a care kit for the new-born to take home. If there were any complications, the woman was taken by ambulance to the nearest hospital for further care. My father was of the belief that one should pay a tiny amount rather than get it all for free. This maintains the self-respect of the individual receiving the treatment and ensures accountability of the service provided.

Choosing the Doctor

Most people choose a hospital that is next door, and then the doctor specializing in the field of concern takes over the patient's treatment. This can be a great option if, financially and logistically, you are limited or just lucky that you have good options close to home!

For others who do not have hospitals and doctors close to home that can provide good quality of treatment, depending on your financial means, it may be beneficial to do some research on good doctors. Sometimes we can have a perfectly good-looking hospital with all the right equipment and state-of-the-art premises, but the doctors may not necessarily be up to date or skilled in the field of treatment.

Things to look for in a doctor:

1) Experience:

    a) The experience of the doctor will give you the satisfaction that he has seen enough patients to know what to expect.

    b) Sometimes you can have a doctor with the best credentials with very little experience and you can have a doctor with maybe not as high credentials but exuberant amounts of experience.

2) Success rate:

a) The success rate will give you insight into the doctor's understanding of the disease and implementation of medical treatment so that you can trust them with your loved one.

b) If there is a doctor with a higher success rate, it is just natural we would want to go to him/her.

c) The problem can be that the more successful and popular a doctor is, the more appointments will be proportionately scarce and harder to get.

3) Reviews:

a) In places like America, Europe and Canada, just like restaurants have YELP ratings, there are ratings available for doctors and hospitals. These are available to the public and you can find them easily.

b) In other countries where these ratings are not available, talk to people around you and see who has had the same medical issue and which doctor treated them. First-hand feedback is the best review one can have!

4) Ease of communication:

a) One of the most important characteristics of a doctor that I like is that the doctor is kind and has 'good bedside' manners, with time to listen and answer your questions in each appointment.

b) Some people like doctors who are more regimental and blunter with little or no empathy for the patient. These doctors usually don't like repeating themselves and answer very briefly, if at all. Their time is limited, so they don't give ample time in consultations for families to ask any questions.

Each person has their own preference, and thank God for that, as we need variety in life. There is always someone for everyone.

If the doctor is easy to talk to and open, there are more chances they will be open to getting a second opinion to make sure they haven't overlooked anything. In some cases, the second opinion doctor will provide alternate treatments which you may or may not want to implement as an addition or primary treatment. This will only be possible if the main doctor is open and willing to incorporate the new treatment into his care.

Half the treatment of the patient happens automatically based on the rapport between the patient and the doctor. This relationship is crucial to the success of the patient's treatment. If the patient is happy to see his/her doctor and feels the empathetic and caring nature of the doctor, the patient will be more likely to go to appointments on time, take the medication happily and overall be more positive and fight harder. Empathy from the doctor, nurses and carers is intrinsic to the patient's care and recovery.

Rights of the Patient (with doctors, hospital, nurses)

The patient is the main actor in this story. Do not forget this! You have to make sure the doctors, nurses, and hospital departments make the patients' benefit the highest priority. Every decision has to take into consideration the patient's comfort, ease, psychological state, physical benefit and overall happiness as the decision-making factors. Nothing, and absolutely nothing, can trump the patient and their requirements. If anybody tries to do or say otherwise, please do not allow them the luxury of overlooking the patient's needs. You must protect the patient if they can't protect themselves.

My mother once had a general doctor overlooking her treatment who was the point of contact for the other specialists in the hospital. For all of you who don't know, once you are admitted to the hospital, most hospitals administer all the medications themselves as they need to monitor the patient very closely. Since my mother had had a full Whipple surgery, she needed insulin administered at every meal and other necessary times depending on the glucose reading. One night before going to sleep at the hospital, her sugar reading was over 300. This is way too much. So I went to the nurse's station and asked the nurse to ask the general doctor how much insulin to administer. The nurse called the doctor in front of me on speakerphone, but the doctor didn't know I was there. The doctor was very rude and impatient and told the nurse, "Why are you disturbing me? My child is crying, and I don't have time for this." I could understand if she was not the main doctor on call to represent the other doctors. I would even understand if she wasn't the doctor on call for my mom specifically. But the fact that she was supposed to be there for my mom and wasn't, really made me mad. Plus, I could have just administered it myself, but I wasn't allowed to do so as per the hospital policy. In any case, we were just lucky that I had gotten my mother's endocrinologist's number (sugar doctor), so I called her directly to ask, and she guided the nurse in administering the right amount of insulin. God bless her!

On the flip side, she was blessed with fantastic doctors in the States who replied almost instantaneously to every question we had. There were two really special doctors she had who flew down and oversaw both her and my dad's progress. One of them was in touch every single day and considered her to be like his mom. Every night, I would send him a summary of the happenings of the day, and by the time I woke up in the morning, he would have replied and told me what to do. With a time difference of 12 hours, this was the norm, but every so often, I would text at a weird time, and he would still answer. Sometimes, I wondered, "Does this human being even sleep?" Once in a while, nothing really important would be going on, so I would skip, and he would say, "Why didn't you write? How is she doing?" He was really special, though, and from the day we met him, he went above and beyond his call of duty to the point where he provided care for so many of my friends and family, too. Doctors like him are godsends, and I pray all of you get doctors like him to guide you. We were extremely blessed to have him in our lives. For me, he was a mentor and a lifeline. I don't know how I would have gotten through caring for my parents without him. He literally would shoot out words at me and expect me to research and figure out what he meant; yeah, he pretty much trained me to be an assistant or a nurse.

Another doctor was her overall oncologist, who never directly treated her, but he made sure he followed all her treatments and approved of what was going on. To this day, we are in touch, and he keeps helping people I know. These amazing doctors are always in our prayers, and we will never forget them for as long as we live.

Medical help

Diagnosis and death are not the only ground-shaking events for terminally ill patients. There are many emergency-inducing situations which will pull the rug out from under your feet. If the patient is diabetic, they can have low sugar-related emergencies.

If they have urine infections, their minds will get confused, and they can start shivering and may even pass out. Blood pressure fluctuations cause all sorts of issues; in some cases, strokes can occur with mismanaged blood pressure and diabetes. Blood pressure and diabetes can cause eye issues, too; in other cases, people have had to get parts of their legs amputated due to uncontrolled diabetes.

Along with these, there are little tricks to consider in the hospital:

1) Comfort of the patient in the hospital

    a) Back of bed and legs in a comfortable position

        i) Keep the pillow to fall behind the top of the back so the head and shoulders are both supported

        ii) Most people will feel more comfortable if there is a pillow under the arm(s)

        iii) Keeping the legs raised is helpful in preventing water retention

    b) If not walking

        i) Blood circulation machine

        ii) Injection to help blood circulation

        iii) Prevent bed sores

        iv) Keep changing their position in the bed

        v) Put powder on their back

        vi) Keep the room aired out and fresh

        vii) Sponge bath

        viii) Massage

Tricks to organise medicine:

1) Make a list of all the medication and their timings

    a) Pills

        i) Pillbox

        ii) Pill cutter

        iii) Get prescription filled on time

    b) Injections

        i) Keep them refrigerated

        ii) Have enough needles at all times

        iii) Make sure to dispose of needles safely

        iv) Rotate the area to inject

        v) Use alcohol swab

        vi) Monitor so that levels don't go too high or too low

    c) Check blood pressure, diabetes, temperature, etc

        i) Make sure you have all the gadgets you need: example - free style libre, glucose, blood pressure monitors, etc.

        ii) Make sure you have all the accessories needed: example - a freestyle libre reader, strips, needles, etc.

2) Keep a diary to record the intake of medication and numbers from monitoring. Also, some machines or accessories have an expiry or need to be changed every so often. For example, the freestyle libre monitor has to be changed every 2 weeks. You must keep at least one extra piece ready.

3) Remember, cortisone or steroids make the sugar go up and cause water retention. They also make the person really hungry so the person will for sure put on weight. They also give a fake

energy high and then the low is really low where the patient will sleep a lot.

4) Remember that fibre cuts sugar. So, if a diabetic person is going to eat sugar, then balance it with some fibre intake. This will keep the sugar from spiking abnormally and also will help their digestive system get rid of toxins.

5) I have found that once a person's immunity is low, as soon as they have high temperatures, chills, brain fog, or such, these are usually signs of some kind of infection. It may be something else, but it is always good to get them checked for infections first.

6) Blood pressure fluctuates:

   a) Static blood pressure can be checked when feeling stressed, tightness in your body, or you feel dizzy. This usually goes high with stress or with excess intake of salts. To bring it down, drink lots of water and try to remain calm.

   b) Orthostatic blood pressure can drop quickly when going from a sitting position to standing. Most commonly, this affects the patient most when getting up from bed in the morning. It is extremely important that the patient learns to slowly turn towards the side of the bed first, then lift their head into a sitting position. They must sit till their body regulates before they stand up. Swift and jerky movements can cause a big drop in blood pressure, which can result in dizziness or a blackout. The patient can faint or fall, causing further complications. Prevention is key!

7) Of course, hydration is very important. Hydrate, hydrate, hydrate! Unless, of course, they are at risk of kidney failure or have ascites or such malady, then their intake of liquids has to

be restricted. One has to be very focused and precise in these situations according to the nature of the illness.

8) Please keep all numbers and email addresses related to treatments and appointments handy and accessible to all carers of the patient.

9) Always keep a bag ready for the hospital with necessary items, including a change of comfortable clothing, toothbrush, toothpaste, grooming kit, shoes, chargers, etc, along with medications and important medical-related gadgets and accessories.

10) Keep all your gadgets charged and ready to go at all times.

If you forget something, remember: you are only human, and humans err all the time. We all do. Don't be hard on yourself. Ask a friend or family member for help. A friend of mine was caring for his mother, and on one occasion, he had to rush his mom to the emergency room, and he left the bag at home. He desperately needed a charger, so he called up his friend in the middle of the night apologetically and asked him to arrange for a charger. The friend was swift in bringing a charger of his own and reassured him that it was an honour to help him and his mother. At the end of the day, that's what friends are for, right? Who knows when he will be in a similar position? Hopefully, he will do the same!

Voice Your Opinions

I think, generally, we people from Asia and Africa put doctors on a pedestal and get scared to discuss, argue or stand up to doctors and nurses. Doctors and nurses are very busy these days, and even if they mean well, most of the time, they are stretched with their time with the volume of patients and each one of their needs. You have to be the voice of the patient with doctors and nurses. In the hospital, from little things like asking for extra pillows and blankets to getting their meds on time or getting the nurses to give the patient a shower or sponge bath. For big things like getting the nurses and doctors to be there for an emergency, like if the patient starts feeling faint or foggy in the brain or shivering, you must press the red button on the bed and run to the nurse's station to get help straight away. Scream and shout if you must without being rude, of course. (Sometimes being rude is the only way to get the right attention, but please do apologise afterwards. They generally understand the panic of loved ones under the stress everyone is worrying about their patients. I learned a great trick: buy them a nice meal right in the beginning and make your mark. This ensures good rapport and a good reputation for yourself to redeem you when you go off-hand!)

I have often wondered about those patients who come there on their own, and for days and days, nobody comes to visit them. How do they get to the washroom without soiling their beds? How long do they have to stay in the soiled sheets? How much pain do they go through when they don't have a pillow under their arm with the ivy needle pulling on their veins in uncomfortable positions? How high does their sugar go after a meal when they have not been given their insulin on time? Or how low does their sugar go when they have been given their insulin ahead of time and they don't eat straight after? If they are at risk of falling, there is an alarm on the beds in some hospitals, so they cannot go to the bathroom without the nurse's permission. The nurses are constantly called for something or another by the many patients on the floor. It is quite understandable that they cannot attend to everyone right away each time. But who knows what kind of dilemmas this causes for each patient?

I don't believe in leaving a loved one at the hospital by themselves.

I understand not everyone has the luxury of being with their loved ones 24/7 at the hospital. Fortunately, I was able to do this with the help of my siblings and others. I am extremely grateful for this. It is so important to have someone with the patient when the doctor comes for his visit to the hospital. The patient isn't always able to retain all the information, and it's always a bonus to have someone else there to take notes or just remember things the patient may forget here and there.

I cannot stress enough that we have to keep the needs of the patient as the number one priority. At this time, nothing can be more important than that. When the needs and comforts of the patient are addressed, the patient can then relax and focus on getting better. If they have to worry about offending the doctor or nurse, they will lose their energy to battle the disease. They have enough pain and other issues to worry about. Why burden them with other unnecessary issues to deal with?

You Know the Patient Best after Him/Herself

When a parent gets sick, it's ideal for the same-sex child to be the carer. There are many private issues, such as changing the catheter, helping in the washroom or shower, aiding the parent to change, etc. This retains the dignity of the patient since, in most cultures, it involves shame to be seen by the opposite sex child. I was fortunate enough to be the carer for both my parents. With my mom, I could do everything from helping her change to helping with washing up needs to changing her wound dressings to holding her while they punctured through her ribcage from the back to put a drain in her lungs to meeting every private issue she may have. With my dad, earlier in life, I was always the one who was there for his stents, his hernia surgery and so on. They were not very intense and didn't require him to be uncomfortable with having me by his side. Later in life, though, it became a bit awkward when I stayed nights with him, and he needed to use a urinal or when he would have discomfort with catheters and the like. However, I ended up changing the catheter bags and learned to handle a bipap machine! By this time, glucose and blood pressure monitors were a regular thing. My point is that my dad would not be comfortable changing in front of me, nor would I be comfortable with that, although I guess when one does not have a choice, you find ways to figure it out. Thank God we were able to get a nurse so he could do all the things I couldn't. This is why I stress that if there is a son, he should take care of the dad, and if there is a daughter, she can take care of the mother. The point is that it's easier to relate to a body that is similar to yours in the case of personal issues which we may not feel comfortable talking to the opposite sex about, especially being your child of the opposite sex.

How to complain in the hospital - when is enough Enough?

This brings us to our next topic for the hospital, what do we do when we have done everything in our hands but the doctors and nurses are not up to par? Do we just stay quiet and accept negligent behaviour and let our patient lose out on their health because we are too shy to complain? Many people may adhere to decorum or societal pressure and say it isn't wise to make a scene. But when your loved one's health is getting affected by someone's mistreatment, then your gut will tell you that it's time to do something about it. Every hospital will have a complaints section or an admin who is responsible for handling HR in the institution. Doctors have an oath they take, it's called the Hippocratic oath, which states in part:

By all that I hold highest, I promise my patients competence, integrity, candour, personal commitment to their best interest, compassion, absolute discretion, and confidentiality within the law...I shall work with my profession to improve the quality of medical care and improve public health, but I shall not let any lesser public or professional consideration interfere with my primary commitment to provide the best and most appropriate care available to each of my patients. To the extent that I live by these precepts, I shall be a worthy physician. (students.med.psu.edu, Penn State University website)

After reading the whole oath, if you feel you have not been done right by the doctors or the institution providing care, you may go ahead and find ways to complain and fix things for your patient's benefit. There is no reason the patient should not get the care he/she deserves to better their health. Normally, there is a CMO (Chief Medical Officer) in the administration who is responsible for assuring that each patient is treated in the best way possible by the staff on every level. The patient cannot fight for themselves, you must fight for them.

CHAPTER 3

DEALING WITH THE PATIENT AND PATIENT REQUIREMENTS

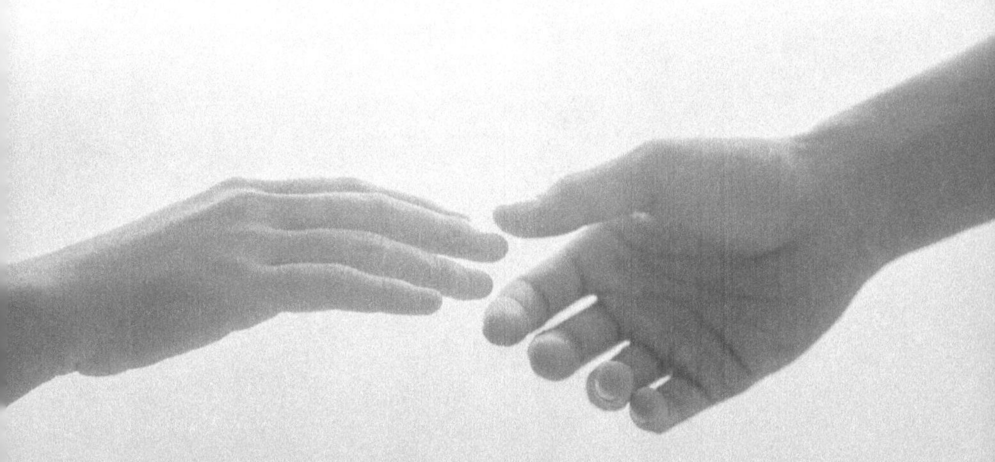

The parent becomes a child, and you become a parent.

When we are children, we depend on our parents for survival - food, drink, clothes, showering, and even our movement is dependent on our parents or whoever is taking care of us. They teach us how to talk and everything we need to know. They pay for our lives even. The key thing is that we do not know anything, and we look to our parents to show us how to live. Now, when they are elderly and sick, they become dependent on us, just like when we were children. Except there is one huge difference, they are used to being in control of their own lives, and they have knowledge and experience way more than you because of their age. To sit back and take directions from you without any of their own input is going to cause friction, and in some cases, the frustration can turn into resentment or hatred.

Let them have control over their life.

It is essential that you, as the carer of your parent, help to preserve the dignity of the parent by allowing them to have control over their life and life decisions. Imagine you lose control over your health: you may or may not be mobile, you can't eat everything you want, your life is dictated by the doctors, and the amount of time you have on earth with your loved ones is limited, and so on. The only control you have would be over the little decisions, including what to wear, what to watch, what to eat, and when to sleep. If you can't even have that much control over your life, then don't you think you will freak out? At times, people choose not to do treatment, but that doesn't mean you have to force them. They are adults, and as long as their mental faculties are intact, let them do what they feel is good for them. We cannot force people to do what we want just because we want it. At the end of the day, it is their life, not ours. We have to give them the space and independence to dictate their life choices, don't we?

Psychological issues

When the patient isn't allowed to exercise their choices freely and face resistance, their emotions may ignite, and they can get angry and stubborn. The mood swings are the result of frustration at not having control over their own lives. This requires the carer to take a step back and separate from the patient and allow them to be the separate entity that they are. It is very important to let the patient retain their psychological balance. Their sanity is your sanity. If their lives are chaotic, then your life will be chaotic too and vice-versa.

Try to remember the quote, even if it's a bit cliche: "Love conquers all." Whatever we do with love always gives fruit. It may take a long time, but if you stick with it long enough, it will undoubtedly give the desired results. Even if the patient gets frustrated and resists your help or care, stay positive and keep reminding yourself of the intention you took on this challenge with. It may sound a bit hocus pocus, but intentions and bringing the higher power into your decisions have a stronger effect than when we do things on our own. When we do it on our own, we are working from the ego.

When we bring in the intention with the Divine, we work from our heart and soul. I truly believe that if we keep focused on our intentions while we give and care for the other, their resistance will succumb to our kindness and good energy.

One example is of a person who had a very tough relationship with her mother. When the mother fell sick, the daughter made a solemn promise to the Divine, namely: "God, I know it pleases you that I take care and be there for my mother. I want to make amends with her, and from now on, I solemnly promise that I will do all that I can to be there for her from the most authentic and genuine part of me, and I will not regress back to who I was around her." From that day forward, she gave all her heart and soul to being there for her mother. It took a year for the mother to understand that it wasn't just situational or fake, but their relationship turned around beautifully. After the one-year mark, they became inseparable and had the most amazing relationship till the mother passed away. It is unfortunate that they wasted so many years having friction between them, but oh well, it's better late than never! Plus, the few years of happiness and love shared between them made the past irrelevant. The good memories are there to look back on to strengthen and comfort her today, long after the mom has left her. There are no regrets.

Regrets are difficult to deal with. Try to fix things now when you can; otherwise, the burdens of these regrets can weigh you down. Death doesn't offer a second chance. When we have not lost a loved one, we don't understand the permanence of losing someone. We don't understand why we are never able to speak to them again. Sometimes, people even miss fighting with the other person. Yet, the saddest part is when we cannot hug and kiss and say 'Sorry' to the person ever again. Try not to let things end without amends.

We don't know who will go first, but either way, no one should be praying for one more chance, wondering what if…?

The patient needs exercise and therapy to deal with fears and anxiety. When we were in Hong Kong, two of the patients came up to my mother and told her that the best treatment for cancer to is to walk for 3 hours a day. Don't stop moving at whatever pace you can. Stop and take a break, but continue. Do not become sedentary, that is destructive. Unfortunately, some of us aren't lucky enough to be able to be mobile when ill, but if you happen to be so blessed, please keep moving!

Exercise helps relieve tension in the body, encourages circulation of blood and oxygen throughout the body, releases endorphins or happy hormones, clears the mind, keeps the muscles strong, lessens fat in the body, and so many other benefits. On the cellular level, exercise diffuses oxygen into the blood cells, and the movement allows the organs to function at their optimum level, helping remove toxins from the body. This can only help the patient become healthier in ways we cannot imagine in addition to the treatments. Nobody is asking the patient to run a marathon, but moving at a comfortable pace throughout the day can only be beneficial to one's health.

The patient will go through a lot of emotional turmoil with fears and anxiety at the helm. There are many options for therapy of, which some include:

1) Therapy

    a) Psychotherapy or Psychiatry

    b) Art therapy

    c) Music Therapy

d) Hypnotherapy

e) NLP

2) Yoga

3) Meditation

4) Crosswords

5) Sudoku

6) Religion - faith

7) Reflexology

8) Reiki

9) Breathwork

10) Energy work

11) Faith-based therapy

Religion brings immense peace to a person going through a life-threatening sickness. The idea that they will be leaving their loved ones to go to an even more loving entity offers a sense of peace and calm to the soul. La illaha illallah = there is nothing other than Allah (God). In Islam, we believe that everything is God, and the act of dying is a sort of 'going back' to the oneness of God. If this is the case, then returning to the most beautiful and kind entity should provide peace and happiness; one should not be afraid to go to God, right? Shouldn't we be happy to reunite with the most merciful and beneficent God? Moreover, in every religion, the concept of dying and reuniting with the most loving entity should be a calming idea devoid of all fear and negativity. For people who believe in a God, it would be of great benefit to speak to their religious representatives. They can guide the patient with prayers which provide solace to the patient's mind and soul.

Many hospitals around the world can organise for a faith-based representative to come to speak to the patient. Most of the time, it is at the end of life that they have a religious representative to prepare the patient for what is to come. Some of us do not have time for this, or we may not want to face the daunting end. If we are connected to a faith-based community or have religious affiliations, we may be able to organise some sessions of our own with a religious guide. Choose wisely, as even in those, there are many ranges, and we do not want the patient to get panicked or stressed more than they already are.

The patient needs entertainment or socialising (outlets)

It's best to organise entertainment or social activities into the patient's schedule. Meeting friends and people of the same age helps the patient feel 'normal'. They can relate at the same level of maturity and share similar issues. Although, I have found that sometimes meeting younger people helps the elderly feel young, included and 'in the know'. Everyone wants to feel needed. Sometimes meeting younger people helps the older ones feel needed and helpful with their advice from their years of experience. My dad loved it when his nephews came and spent time with him to discuss work-related issues over a nice meal in his favourite restaurant or cafe. He loved that people still took his advice for work since he was still working for a few hours a day at the age of 82! He loved it even more when they took him out to watch a cricket game or concert. My mom and dad enjoyed life tremendously. Their zest for life included watching movies, going to restaurants, travelling, and attending shows of all kinds - pretty much everything I do reminds me of them as they partook in all the activities with us and more! I hope and pray I can enjoy life all the way to my grave like them. It kept them young and gave them that extra fight to live life longer than the odds.

As the doctor once told my mother - Don't make cancer your life! Cancer or other illnesses are a part of your life, not your whole life. Focus on maintaining a life other than the disease for the patient. We pray and beg God to give us a longer life, but maybe God is asking us, "What are you doing with the life that I am giving you now?" Show him what you can do with the extra time, and if it's worthy enough, he may just give you more. If not, at least you are getting done what you need to, and hopefully, you are training someone in the process to continue the good work that you do!

This is a very tough concept to implement, indeed. Many patients undergo relentless treatment, which doesn't afford them the luxury of continuing to be involved in their day-to-day activities in their regular fashion. Yet, one should try to be the parent, friend, lover, boss, employee, or whatever other role one plays in one's pre-illness life. So many theories these days encourage controlling the mind and projecting the future in an ideal way to manifest other than what is at the moment. When done properly, miracles take place, and so it is worth the effort. Whether one succeeds or not, at least the mind is positive, and the patient will have respite from their pain and situation by imagining a disease-free life and doing their 'normal' activities.

Physical challenges

A very important issue to be aware of, and I cannot stress this enough, is trying to prevent the patient from falling at whatever cost. Falling after a certain age can be disastrous. I have seen way too many people fall and hurt their hips, and their decline starts fairly quickly after that. Surgeries in late ages take forever to heal. Anaesthesia is harder to handle with other complications and age-related diseases. With diabetes, healing is even harder or impossible sometimes. Bones become brittle and are easier to crack. If your heart is weak, the surgeries can be very tough to endure. With osteoporosis, any type of fall can be extremely dangerous to all your bones, especially the lower spine.

It is imperative that a patient uses aids when they start to feel unbalanced:

1) Wheelchair

2) Walking Stick

3) Walker

4) Rollator walker with a seat to rest and a place to keep belongings

5) Hearing aids and glasses

6) Hospital bed

7) Brace for osteoporosis fracture L1 & L2

So, we all don't like to feel dependent on aids, and our egos prevent us from using gadgets. It hurts our pride to sit in a wheelchair or use a walking stick. I get it. I tore my Achilles tendon when I was 22 years old and had a cast from the top of my thigh to my foot, but I refused to sit in a wheelchair. Every week for 6 weeks, the doctor would come home to see me, and I would ask him, "Doctor, will I be able to walk again?" And every week, he would look down and humbly say, "I don't know." I was so stubborn I refused to sit in a wheelchair. I got someone to hold my leg in the air walking backwards while I walked with crutches forwards. The person could have tripped walking backwards and hurt themselves, which would have caused me to fall and break more parts of my body and undo all the effort that the operation had done. How stupid, inconsiderate, and selfish was I? I could have hurt others and myself. Wouldn't it have been better and safer to just sit in the wheelchair with my leg up and have someone push me? I don't know, but just looking at that wheelchair, the thought of being bound to it for life freaked me out. I think I sat on it twice because there was no other way to get to the place. Sometimes, I feel that the reason I am walking and running today is that I just didn't accept that I wouldn't walk. There was no choice for fate or God or anything to make me succumb to that option. So maybe that's how most people feel, and it prolongs the need to depend on a mobility aid. But a fall in that situation would have ruined everything, I am just lucky I didn't fall.

It's the same when we get older. Our pride and ego don't allow us to use that walking stick or walker even though we feel our body getting imbalanced. We may even reach out for the railing on the staircase or reach out for a hand at the time we feel imbalanced, but we will not tarnish our reputation of being 'young and fit'. There is a block in our heads to 'need' an apparatus for mobility. Have you thought of the alternative? Imagine you do not use the seat in the shower or the walking stick in the park, and in the blink of an eye, you slip and find yourself on your back, not able to move. They rush you to the hospital, and now you have fractured your hip or your back. The doctor says you will be bedridden until the fractures heal. Or you might need hip surgery or knee surgery. These are two very painful surgeries, and for the elderly, it can be very hard to heal, taking way longer than the average person. The nurses cannot move you around, so you are stuck sleeping in the same position for days. You start getting bed sores, and after a while, they are out of control. It could turn into a life-threatening situation, or worse, it could require an appendage to be amputated. Wouldn't it just be better and easier for everyone to use the walking stick or walker or wheelchair? Isn't quality and quantity of life both better with some help?

DEALING WITH THE OTHER PARENT

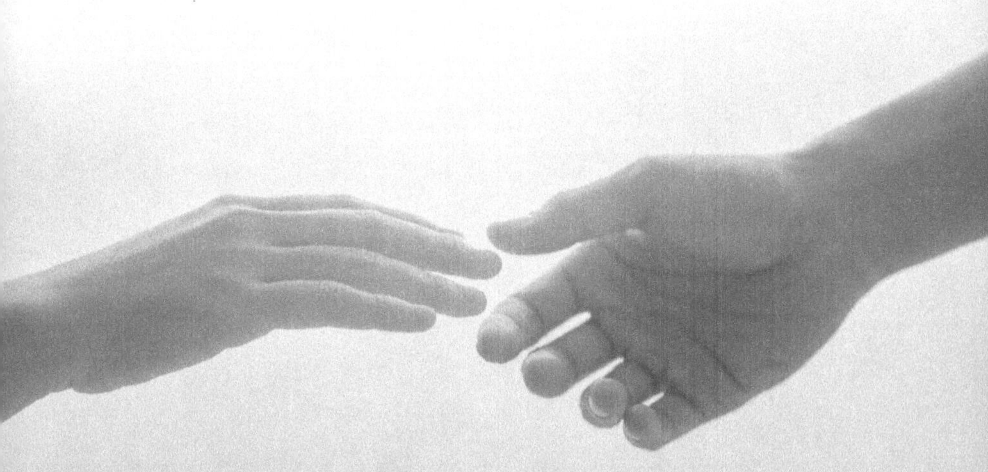

Needs attention

The other parent or spouse of the patient may or may not be able to be the carer. They cannot be forgotten in the process if they are not the main carer. If they are not able to care for their spouse, then they might need caring also. We have to remember to make sure they are taking care of their health with proper food and exercise. We do not want them to end up getting sick, either. Imagine having 10 pills to take in the morning and another 10 scattered throughout the day - that's for the patient. Now, think about all the appointments and extra information regarding the patient one has to remember. If the spouse is the carer, imagine where their own meds and nutrition must be on the list. Luckily, if the spouse is not the main carer, they will still try to be able to keep up with their spouse's schedule and needs. But imagine if they are old and have a bunch of meds and appointments of their own?

The spouse will also need extra attention to feel special, as they may feel redundant and useless. It is vital that they are given some importance so as to feel like they are useful. As their partner is not able to do what they used to, the spouse is left in limbo as concerns their well-being emotionally (no one to talk to about personal and family issues), psychologically (talking through issues) and sometimes physically (food-wise). This can leave the spouse extremely vulnerable, or it may make them bitter and hard to handle. It can go either way.

Needs to have control

The other parent has to be part of the decision-making process to feel important and useful. Remember, till the day before the diagnosis, the parents were the ones who enjoyed their privacy, made all the decisions for themselves and had control over their lives. Now, all of a sudden, their lives are in an upheaval, and there is no privacy or control. The ill parent has to share all their information with the family, but even the other parent has you and the rest of the family coming in and out of the house and their lives more often than they are used to. Even if we are their kids, for us to tell them what to do and what not to do, move stuff around in the house, dictate how and when appointments will be made, which accessories to put around the house for the disabled parent, and so many other decisions, cause a lot of havoc and will throw them off. In these cases, we must be patient and make the changes slowly and even better, try to make it sound like their idea rather than yours. People accept change way better when they think they decide to make the changes themselves rather than listening to others.

The spouse of the patient is not sick, and they are just as capable as they were before they found out about the illness. The only difference is that they are now emotionally affected, and that emotional impact will present itself in many surprising ways. As strong as they may be, they will be shattered, and the emotional instability will affect their decision-making abilities. The brain fog will hinder their understanding of the medical jargon doctors throw at them. Sometimes, even if they understand English, if it is not their first language, they will find it challenging to comprehend the complexity of the situation and the details of the disease with its protocol. All these issues will require you to be their interpreter and liaison with the doctors and nurses. You will need to be extremely patient and allow time for the information to sink in so they can calmly make decisions or at least give their input. The danger of them not being able to be part of the process is that later, when the fog lifts, they may blame you for things that may have gone wrong, and you definitely don't want that! After all, it is the patient's life first, and that life is most precious to the spouse before the children.

They use you as their boxing bag to vent

Also, usually, couples depend on each other for emotional support and to vent on each other. Since their partner is now sick, they will not want to burden them with their own problems. The person or child who is the carer for the ill parent will spend the most time with the parent who is healthy. The frustrations and mood swings the healthy parent feels will not be addressed to the ill spouse anymore, as they will not want to burden them at this time. Consequently, the caregiver will become the boxing bag, as the famous adage goes: "We fight with the ones who love us or who we are around the most." Be ready; they have a lot to deal with, having their closest person fighting for their lives. Nobody has a handbook, and nobody prepares for these things; we learn on the job. There will be a lot of ups and downs. They will have tons of unanswered questions and worries. The future is so uncertain that they will lose all composure and control, which will inevitably come out in all kinds of ways.

Be patient and kind, and when you can't be, take some time

out. Do something to bring you back to a good place inside and make you stronger. Try to stay in the present, meditate and at that time, in that second, ask yourself: "Would I want to be anywhere else other than taking care of the parent who is sick? How would I be if my spouse was going through a terminal illness? Would I be nice all the time, or would I need a punching bag too?" If you are completely true to yourself at that moment, you will see that you would not be able to handle the situation any better than your parents, considering their age.

Health needs

As we age, we get accustomed to our routines getting set in our ways. Eventually, we start losing our balance, our body parts ache constantly, our reflexes slow down, our brain becomes foggy, and we start getting issues like blood pressure, diabetes, cholesterol, arthritis, migraines, back pain, osteoporosis, hard of hearing or deafness, sight problems, and the list goes on and on. Our parents show us the way in which our genetics will influence what we get from them. What they are going through, we will go through some, if not all, the issues. So try to imagine, if you had what they have, how would you behave? Would you complain? Would you be short-fused? Would you be able to gracefully tolerate all that your parents are going through?

The best way to create harmony is to continue looking after their health care and needs. The more the spouse stays healthy and independent, the longer they will live, and you won't have to take care of both of them at the same time. Yes, they can both need carers at the same time. My mother was going through bile duct cancer treatment when my dad was diagnosed with bladder cancer. Bladder cancer, if the tumour goes into the bloodstream, is game over unless you undergo surgery to remove the bladder and restructure it. At the age my dad was at the time, there was no chance he would survive such a surgery. We were extremely fortunate that his tumour grew inward and didn't advance into his muscle tissue or bloodstream. Thank God! The best thing was he never even believed he had cancer, although it was for sure that the tumour was malignant, and he went through many cystoscopies to follow up. God bless his soul, he lived for 6 years after he was diagnosed and passed away in his sleep peacefully five years after my mother, God bless her soul.

We thought it was tough enough to be caring for one parent, but imagine having both parents in two separate hospitals, needing you to be there for all the doctors' visits to understand each of their situations. Thank God we are five siblings! Although we don't all live in the same city, out of sheer luck of fortune, all of us were in town for this event, so we shared the caregiving. I have never been so happy to have so many brothers and sisters, haha! I bet the parents were grateful beyond words, too, that they had their battalion of kids. At this point, I felt really sorry for the people who had just 1 or 2 kids!

Emotional support

The spouse needs emotional support and lots of it. First of all, they have lost their everyday support; clearly, they wouldn't want to be burdening the ill parent with their issues. Rather, the spouse now has to support the ill spouse more to ease their pain and worries. For their own support, they will turn to the children, which will take a lot of getting used to for them and for you and your siblings. So, try to remember the other parent and give them love, affection, and hugs. Every human needs physical touch and knowing people care. A 20-second hug is known to be therapeutic and curative. "A 20-second hug reduces harmful effects of stress, relieves blood pressure, and ensures a healthy heart. Increasing the hug ratio results in reduced blood pressure, decreased cortisol, improved healing, reduced cravings and better immunity." (https://www.medicinenet.com/how_do_hugs_make_you_feel) Tracy P. Alloway, PhD, describes experiments done to prove the benefits of hugs. She further explains that it's not the number of hugs that counts; it's the length of the hug that matters the most. (www.psychologytoday..com/us/blog/keep-it-in-mind/202201/what-20-seconds-hugging-can-do-you)

My mom was always affectionate, and everyone who knows her has had her signature 'tight hug'. My dad and the rest of us kids were not so physically affectionate. Yet, when my mom got sick, she insisted on giving everyone a 'tight hug' and an 'I love you' before she went to sleep. It helped her and us, and we all got used to it. Now I miss those, I got used to it. Why do we resist things that are good for us? Especially when deep down inside, we all need love and care regardless of who we are.

Support group

Since they need to vent and talk through their situation, it's best to find your non-sick parent, a support group, a therapist or help them make a schedule that incorporates interacting with their friends. We have to understand that their best friend is sick and not available to hear their everyday issues. They cannot even talk to their spouse about how they are feeling - scared, worried, etc about the sick spouse. Men, especially in the Global South and Eastern part of the world, will close up and have difficulty communicating their feelings. Men have been taught since they were young: be strong, don't cry, don't talk about your feelings, be the fixer, have all the answers, and so on. Women, on the other hand, can generally cry more easily and have a friend or more to relay their feelings to get their dose of therapy. Women are more likely to get included in activities or will make tea or lunch happen to meet friends and relieve their chest of worries and insecurities. Men are not so open with their feelings and are more likely to keep everything bottled up. If anything, in their free time, they will get themselves busy with their work. If they are able to play a sport or other physical activity, that will be really good for them to release the tension in their body. For both, a good massage or long soak in the tub would be magnificent.

Even at their age, they will need to be strong to support their ill spouse. Naturally, they will try to be extra nice to the ill spouse, so all their venting and frustration will need to be addressed elsewhere. Usually, we dump our misery on the closest person. Unfortunately, you will be that person and the target of all frustration. Everything will be your fault and will be treated as a dump truck for anger and moodiness. Be strong and understanding. I know your plate is full, and you are under a lot of pressure but try to take a step back and see the situation for what it is. Connect with God again, indulge in your meditative practices, and you will see you are stronger than you think! You can handle it all with the help of spiritual guidance. Besides, it's not you they are angry at, they are just frustrated with the situation and don't know what else to do.

Nutrition and supplements - food

While our focus is completely on the patient, the spouse's nutritional needs can easily be overlooked. This is not acceptable as they are also fragile, and their needs have to be met to prevent them from falling ill. Their nutrition - fresh food that supports their medical requirements- has to be prepared to ensure longevity in their life. Supplements are also very important, such as vitamins, which need to be bought and refilled if running out. The lack of vitamins like vitamin D, vitamin C and magnesium may be related to of the progression of illnesses such as osteoporosis, arthritis, diabetes, and others. To ensure that their health stays stable, it is best to keep such details updated.

Try to keep them away from sugar although it helps psychologically for emotional eating but at the end of the day you crash in energy. They say tumours love sugar like us and they grow faster with sweet stuff. Best is to grow or retain muscle since muscle eats fat and carbs. One generally doesn't need extra sugar as it is released anyway from most foods even if you don't eat it. The extra carbs and fat we eat release sugar or glucose that we need, and the rest is stored as fat. Nobody needs extra fat do we? So continue strength training and let the muscles do what they should be doing and stay healthy!

Friction in relationships

I have spoken to many people who have gone through a similar experience. Most people voice concerns about the many conflicts that ensue between siblings during the process of taking care of their parents. We all get emotional and sensitive when our parents get sick. All the siblings, in their own way, are affected and get easily frustrated or angry. We want to protect the ill parent, plus we want to take care of them, yet we can't be present physically all the time. When we cannot physically take care of the parent, we tend to control the situation with our advice and opinions. It's lovely to participate, and the carer definitely needs support from the siblings, but be respectful of the fact that the carer is in charge. If the patient gets serious or sicker, it is the carer who will have to put in the extra time and assume the umpteen responsibilities to follow - so please respect the carer and don't do things without telling him/her - it's not a competition! At this time, we need to come together as a team. Work together - things will be so much easier for everybody. If you perform as a team, the parents will be happy; all parents' dream is to see their children get along, whatever age they are. Unity in the family reflects the unity of the divine. When we fight, we not only hurt our parents, but we also hurt God. If both the parents and God are happy, the results will always be good.

Feelings of abandonment and uselessness

It is very easy for a healthy spouse to get ignored and forgotten. In the hustle and bustle of taking care of the patient, the whole family's focus is concentrated on the patient. Between their medicine, hospital visits and other needs, the other parent gets side-lined unintentionally. When this happens, that parent, just like anyone else, will feel abandoned and useless. You have to remember that this person has spent their entire married life taking care of the spouse and preserving their privacy. Now, all of a sudden, the ill parent is the only one that matters. The crazy thing is that the other parent wants the ill parent to be taken care of, but at the same time, they need attention, too. This creates a dichotomy that can instigate feelings of insecurity and vulnerability, which can easily turn to anger and meanness as a defence mechanism. If they continue to be ignored and they aren't very expressive or vocal about their feelings, they could possibly go into depression.

One of the ways to prevent this catastrophe is to remember

that we are all children at the end of the day. If we learn to forgive our parents and siblings as easily as we forgive our own children, only then will we be able to keep the peace and harmony of our family unit intact. Why is it so easy to forgive our own children but impossible to forgive other people who are the children of God? Someone once told me that the best way to have more patience and understanding with others is to imagine them as children while talking to them. It works like a charm!

Fear of being alone after and grief

It's almost like the spouses lose their other half two times: once while the patient is alive and second when they pass. The grief they live with while either taking care of their spouse or just watching the spouse suffer must be intolerable. We can never truly understand what someone goes through until we go through it ourselves, but we can try to empathise with them and feel for them. Therefore, we may learn to forgive them for their callousness. When we try to understand another's position, it makes us feel soft towards them, and it makes it easier to be patient and forgiving. Be kind to the parent going through their grief. Try to communicate more with them and get them to talk about it. Sometimes, it's not easy to talk about it, so just let them know you are there. Words are not always necessary. Most of the time we just need to know that the other person cares and is there for us whatever it takes.

CHAPTER 5

DEALING WITH YOUR SIBLINGS

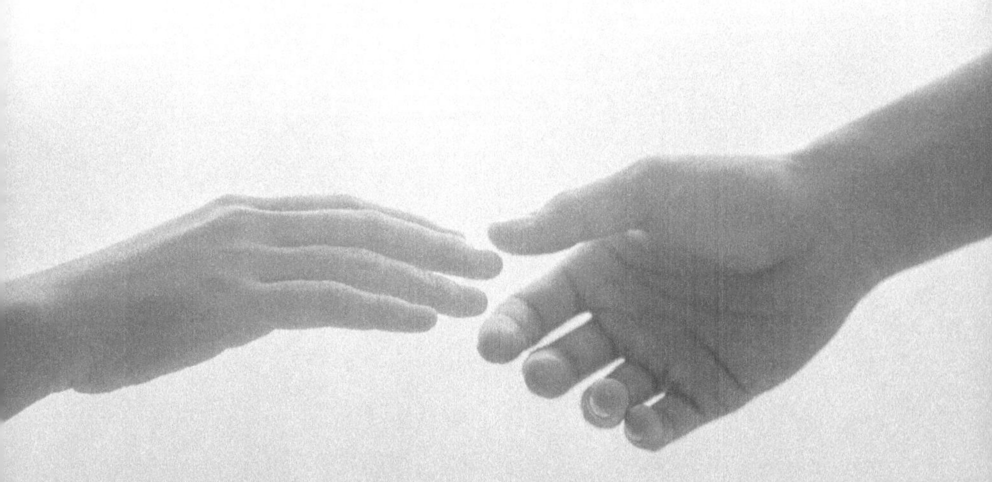

Sharing responsibilities

Delegating responsibilities to others, especially your siblings, is crucial. The responsibility of a parent's life can be a tremendous task that can only be shared with your siblings. The load will never be evenly distributed, but knowing that all are putting in time and effort will provide peace to all, especially the parents. Parents love it when their kids (whatever age they may be, will always be kids to them) take time out of their lives to take care of their parents. This is love that is almost equal to the parent taking care of the child. It can never be equal because they had to take care of one or more children physically, emotionally, and financially, giving of their own physical, emotional and financial capabilities.

Think about the big decisions, such as surgeries, treatments and such, when they go wrong, do you want to be the sole decision-maker at that time? Do you want to take full responsibility for things if they go wrong? Do you want to take the chance of making decisions when you are clearly not a connoisseur or learned enough in this field to take the responsibility of making decisions for the life of someone so dear to you? When we share responsibilities, we ensure an equal distribution of responsibility for care, decision-making and love for the patient between all the siblings. This prevents blaming and finger-pointing in the event that something goes wrong. It also lets the parent know that they are loved by all equally and everyone gets to display their loving care in their own capacity. The respect of each member is thus retained - intact, or may even grow positively in this way.

You will, in essence, become the parent of your sick parent overnight. This is no small feat. Parents are naturally self-sufficient and decision-makers handling their own lives to an extent. All of a sudden, being put in charge of a parent's life can be a huge challenge and, in some cases, traumatic.

Decision-making clashes

The decision-making process can prove to be extremely challenging. We are as human beings very different in our ways of thinking and doing things. If any situation will display this, it is when a parent is ill. Everyone thinks they are right or that they know best. All of a sudden, the parents seem like they are not sure of themselves, and each kid will try to push their ideas on them like it's some kind of competition.

Competition

Discord with parents and siblings or any other close family member at this time is inevitable. Everyone is high-strung, and emotions are bouncing, it is only natural that we are the most sensitive and susceptible at this time. Some may become extra competitive by nature, others may just disappear under pressure, and yet others will become critical of every step without putting in the effort. The best thing is to take a step back and take time out for yourself so that when you come back to the situation, you can see it more objectively.

Guilt issues

Depending on the sibling relationship, there can be guilt put on each other for not doing enough. In other cases, they can put blame on each other if something were to go wrong, big or little. For example, if there are choices to be made to do a treatment at a certain time, but one person decides to do it later, and things go out of hand in the meantime, then fingers might be raised.

It is extremely important in these cases to remember that fate is orchestrating the overall play of things. We can only make decisions to the best of our knowledge at the time, the rest is up to God's will and the fate of the patient. We cannot fall into the guilt trap, nor can we throw others into it. Every step of the way, one has to remember God and His wisdom. We are not in control as much as we like to think we are. We do what we can, and God decides the outcome.

Blame Game

Everyone is high-strung and overly sensitive at this time. On the other hand, some will become extra selfish when they are used to getting all the attention from their parents, and now they can't get it. When things go wrong, it is very easy to blame the other. It will be very easy to blame each other for stupid reasons, or it could be for big, important reasons like:

1) Missing appointments: Nobody misses appointments on purpose, but it could happen that the calendar gets confused or, an email gets missed, and an appointment gets overlooked. Yes, it can be very stressful and scary, but doctors are usually very understanding. If the doctor doesn't understand, then hopefully, the secretary or nurse will be kind enough to understand and will rebook it as soon as possible.

2) Mishaps like the patient taking a fall: Accidents are not planned; they just happen, and that's why they are called 'accidents'. It isn't anyone's fault, and there is no point in assessing what could have or should have been done. Accept that it happened and do what is necessary moving forward.

3) Sugar reading going high: There are many reasons for the sugar level spiking in an individual. Yes, eating sugary foods does make it spike, but stress can make it spike, too. The sweet treats the patient eats can be balanced by eating some fibre. Fibre helps keep the sugar levels from spiking. So, if your patient feels like having a treat here or there, just give them some fibre and let it be. For stress-related spikes, one has to engage in some kind of exercise or stress-reducing meditations or activities.

4) Surgery aftermath gets complicated: Not all surgeries will go as planned. Many times, the aftermath of the surgery or treatment is more difficult than the surgery itself. My mother's Whipple's surgery took about 6 hours, and she had an incision from her chest to her lower abdomen. To top it off, the cut was deep and left open to heal in its time. Naturally, it required her to get the dressing changed a couple of times a day. The wound kept getting infected and, at times, would heal from the top and not the inside. One such time, the doctor came in and started cutting her wound area, where the skin was numb after the surgery. Crazy! Eventually, she had to get a wound VAC, and then only did she heal properly. Anyway, the point is that she was supposed to recover within a month or 6 weeks, but it took much longer, which pushed back the radiation treatment she was meant to receive. We can't control everything. We can just do our best in every situation.

5) Decisions are made, then regretted because something goes wrong, but nobody is ready to take the blame: At this point, everyone will blame the person in charge, that is you! Whether it is your fault or not, you will be the one they point fingers at because it's easy, and nobody likes to have the burden of guilt or remorse when making bad decisions for their loved ones.

6) While the patient is going through treatments, everyone's brains will be in a fog. It will work well for what you need it to work, but when one looks back at the time, it is very hard to remember exactly what happened. After a good friend's parent passed away, the spouse, in their grief, blamed the carer child for a bad decision that they believed instigated complications in the treatment, leading to the premature death of their ill spouse. When that parent finally voiced their concern to their offspring 6 months later, the son could finally remind the parent of the exact happenings at that time. It turns out all the decisions made at that time were the parents and the other siblings, not the carer's. The doctors had insisted on one decision, and the carer had agreed, but the rest of the family wanted to move since they were missing family and a 'homelike' feeling.

7) The biggest issues happen after the patient, unfortunately, passes away after trying everything. These can be caused by:

   a) Regrets of not having done enough because of:

      i) Distance issues

      ii) Other responsibilities

      iii) Burnout

   b) Not having spent enough time with the ill parent.

   c) Not being involved enough in the decision-making and/or appointments.

d) Comparing and competing for accolades in society.

Being the main carer and decision-maker, you will be the first one to get your fingers pointed at because you were the one to make the ultimate decisions. This is a natural by-product of the responsibility you have undertaken. When you decide to be a carer, be prepared. You will be grieving too and will have all the pressures everyone else has, but this will be another added challenge you will have to deal with. The aftermath gets very complicated when there are issues like wills and inheritances involved; everyone gets even more selfish with their grief and regrets, and things can get nasty, rooted in the pain and anger everyone is feeling at that point. As a family, try to communicate your feelings and needs as much as you can. Communication and making yourself vulnerable are the keys to good relationships. You must stay strong at this point and remember that, ultimately, everything that happened had a reason to happen the way it did. We can plan and do as much as we can, at the end of the day, God's plan is what will triumph. As they say, "Everything is as it should be." We may not understand it logically or with our limited human capacity, but life happens with the consent of the Higher Power. We can only do our best and leave the rest up to Him. He will take care of you now, too, as He took care of everything before.

Too much advice from others - pros and cons

On the other hand, when people give too much advice and are trying to micromanage you, you need to set up boundaries. Also, when they give a huge list of alternatives, it may not be possible for you to implement that into the patient's regime. Or the patient may not be able to actually ingest so many different items during the day. We then have to prioritise the medicines and herbs, etc, and give the patient what they want and only add the most important sounding extra treatments. It will be a tough call, but it is better than frustrating the patient by giving them all of it or by short-changing the patient by denying them of it. This is the time to research and figure out which are the more preferred and effective choices of additional treatment.

Advice from others is good, don't get me wrong. Sometimes, they tell us which herbs or medicines to take in addition to the treatment. Others will share their experiences, and we will learn what is good and what is bad for the patient. Their experiences in the hospitals can give us insight into what to expect from the doctors, nurses, treatments, etc. These are all very good when done with good intentions from both sides. Most people who have been through these difficult situations are very helpful and always eager to help in whatever way they can. Lean on the ones you can, ignore the others. That's life, isn't it?

Can share experiences

The more we share our experiences with others, the more people will open up about theirs. This can be a blessing, lending insight into what to expect and what to avoid. You can also compare experiences along the way. Having someone who can understand what you are going through and relate on the same level is a huge bonus, cherish it! Most of the time, you will feel like nobody can understand you or that you are living on a separate planet from the rest of the world. Anyone who can empathise or relate in any way will be more than welcome in your life right now. Siblings would be the easiest people to connect with since they are also involved in the parent's treatment and can potentially relate most to what you are going through.

Sometimes, when we open up to others, they start crying to us about their own problems irrelevant to what you are going through. Seriously??! You would think they would have more sense and empathy than that, but trust me people can be extremely self-centred and egotistical. They can make anything about themselves. Be prepared, try not to get too shocked, make an excuse and walk the hell away!

Help each other with doctors and nurses.

The best way to go about handling this situation to which you are new at is to communicate with your siblings. When the appointments and talks with doctors and nurses get complicated, discuss openly with each other. Yes, there will be friction, and yes, everyone will have their opinions, but sometimes talking about things makes for clearer and well thought-out decisions. Plus, it is always better that everyone has a say in the decision-making process. After all, the parent is everyone's parent, not just yours.

We may tend to get possessive with the care of the parent, it is only natural. It is a huge responsibility, and one must take it seriously and commit fully to it. On the other hand, please try to remember that the parent loves each child unconditionally and has varied ways of connecting with them. Since each one of you is different, the thinking process and handling of situations will be different, too. Try not to judge each other. The parents will be happy with each of your ways of doing things even though you may think your way is the only way that is right. When you need a break, leave a schedule and explain the important measures to be taken, then let it go. Everyone is an adult and needs their autonomy. The parent and the child will do what they do, you will only lose sleep and stress for nothing. You cannot control others. Trust in the One above and go have a good time, checking in every so often to ask them if they need anything. Most likely, they won't since everyone has their ego and won't want to show their insecurities. When you go back, you can resume your style of caring, in the meantime, get some rest and relaxation. You will find it's a great way to refuel. Boy, do you need it!

Usually, when you take that break, you will end up falling sick. All the stress from the responsibility and happenings gives you an adrenaline rush while you are in caring mode. Once you relax, the body lets go and signals to release everything it has been holding on to. Most of the time, this will result in you getting a fever, flu or infection of some kind. I feel it's the body's way of asking for attention since you have been ignoring yourself. Take this time to spoil yourself and get all the rest you need. You may not feel it, but you deserve all the care and attention you give to others for yourself. Be kind to yourself, and remember: you are only human!

CHAPTER 6

HANDLING INSURANCE ISSUES

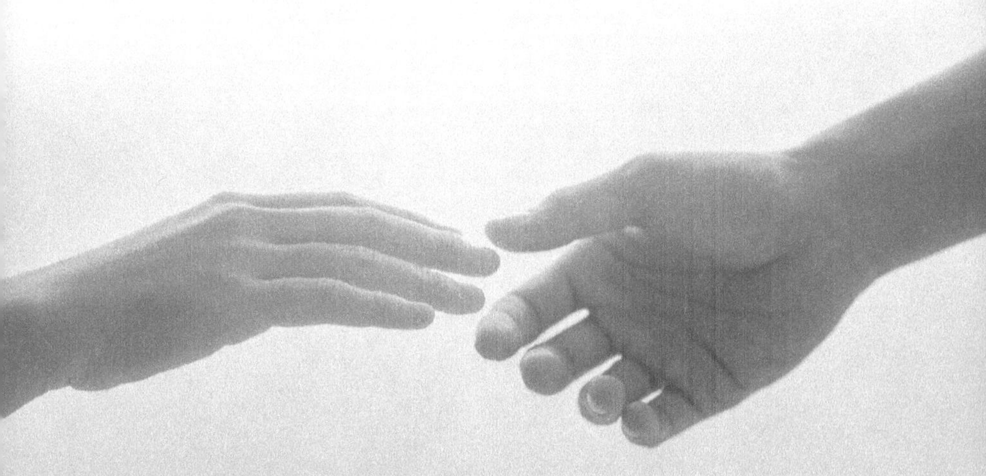

H**ave insurance or not?**

We all are going to get sick one day or the other. It's a reality we all have to face, some early on and others when we get older. But, the truth is, some time or another, we are going to have to go in for surgery or treatment or some procedure that is going to cost us an arm and a leg. It is inevitable except for the fortunate few who are so healthy they never need to go to the hospital and then pass away peacefully in old age. These few make up a handful of people probably in the world. I do not know anyone personally who has been so fortunate.

Pre-existing conditions, usually 1 or 2 years of no pay

For the rest of us 'normal' human beings, we need to prepare financially for such events. Some people complain that paying for health insurance when one is healthy is a waste of money. Well, first of all, do we know when we are going to get sick? These things don't come with warnings, and by the time we get sick, the insurance companies are smart; they charge premiums once you are sick. Others do not cover 'pre-existing' conditions for a year or two, and others never cover pre-existing conditions at all. Furthermore, they don't even cover conditions that can be instigated by the pre-existing conditions you have. This creates a huge dilemma because it is only the luck of the draw that you get diseases or accidents that happen for which you can afford the treatment.

In the USA, if you pay outright for, let's say, a simple appendix operation, it can cost in the 10's of thousands of dollars. In third-world countries, it would be a quarter of the price. Compared to each one's standard of living and labour costs, both prices are exorbitant. These health issues can cause humongous dents in people's budgets out of the blue and create upheaval in people's lives. Wouldn't it be better to pay little by little every month toward, God forbid, anything happening in the future? The money is recovered pretty quickly, as hospitals have a beautiful, sneaky way of adding up the costs of treatment once you are in there. They are a profit-making business most of the time, after all.

Secondly, this is one of the only expenditures in your life that you pray you don't have to use. One should be extremely grateful if one doesn't get a chance to make use of the money we pay for health insurance. Also, God forbid one does get cancer or is in a disastrous accident; all the money one has put towards health insurance will be recovered very easily. So, even if you are the best businessman in the world, the ROI for paying for health insurance is a win-win situation for the individual. It can either be thought of as a 'sadaqah' (charity) that will ward off evil or bad things from happening or if you actually get sick, then your investment will only reap benefits for you financially.

Pros and Cons of Insurance

On the flip side, if you don't get health insurance, yes, you will save a chunk of money because the cost of insurance per person in the family is quite hefty. Of course, it might be a good idea to get health insurance starting from, let's say, 50 years of age, as that is around the mark when everyone's bodies slow down a bit. Some people don't get it at that time either as they may be really fit, exercise, and eat healthy, so they don't get the most common illnesses like diabetes, high blood pressure, or cholesterol. Yet, have we not all heard of young people getting into debilitating accidents, needing surgeries and spending days, if not months, in the hospital? Cancer doesn't have an age limit, does it? We have all heard of the young children at our children's hospitals getting treatments and some having to spend days or months in the hospitals. In Canada and the USA, they have cinemas and play areas in the children's hospitals so that they feel homely and comfortable for the long periods of time they have to spend there.

When we haven't had to deal with hospitals and insurance and illnesses, we think it's all very simple. We think everything is like a broken bone, put on a plaster or cast and go home with crutches or a sling. Or get an appendix or hernia removed, stay one-night maximum in the regular hospital room and go home with crutches. It is not that simple and easy.

In-patient or Out-patient coverage or both?

Do you know how expensive a surgery can be in the USA or in Canada if you don't have OHIP or in the UK if you don't have NHS coverage? Something that costs maybe a couple of thousand US Dollars in third-world countries can cost tens of thousands of dollars in the US. Do you know how expensive it is to be in the ICU for a night anywhere in the world compared to a regular room if you don't have some kind of health insurance? It can cost up to two or three thousand dollars per night for ICU care. In third-world countries, it is proportionally lower, but compared to the cost of living, it can be an obscene amount.

That is just the 'in-patient' cost. Then we have 'out-patient costs', which include things like consultations, emergency room visits that are less than a certain amount of hours, non-prescription medicines and in other cases, even prescription medicines and home care, the list goes on. Then you have MRI, CT Scan, PET scan and other major tests, like DNA tests for tumours and even some blood tests, which can be exuberantly priced. So we think, ok, these are things we have to do, so we will figure out how to pay for these and maybe ask the hospitals to give a discount because most hospitals do have concessions for people who don't have insurance and are paying out of pocket. Ok, so cool. You got your discount, and everything is good.

But now, the patient needs 24/7 care, and you all work and the kids are at school. No one is home to help the patient shower, cook, clean, administer medicine and give them company. You now may need to get a nurse or hire a helper. If you are lucky and live in the West, you may be able to get a social worker to come home a few hours a day to help with these activities. But even those countries are overwhelmed with their public health care systems, and it's so difficult to qualify, and the time is so limited that they have to give to each patient in their homes.

When we go abroad to get treatment, we need to pay for a place to live while getting treatment. In many parts of the world, there is a charitable foundation called Ronald McDonald House Charities (RMHC) that offers housing for such families. They help as much as they can with food, essentials, a place to stay, support from other families and volunteer staff, and even a little bit of schooling for children during the stay, all for a little or no cost. Travel expenditures are at a minimum because the location of these charitable houses is always near the acclaimed hospitals or clinics. It is a beautiful option to look into as I know first-hand that they deliver as per their word. They are an amazing organisation with their motto being: "We believe that 'home' is more than four walls and a roof over your head. That's why every Ronald McDonald House is a safe haven that provides all the comforts of home, plus the compassion and hospitality of staff, volunteers, and other families - all just steps away from the hospital." (rmhc.org)

Many countries around the world have hospices for palliative care treatment for patients, which are free or at a low cost. Treatments for kidney care and other such illnesses may also be available at low costs or for free. Many hospitals have welfare or international departments which allow for discounts. Please ask, there is no harm in asking. The worst that can happen is they say 'No.' but what if they say 'Yes!'? The amount of money treatments and procedures cost, it's always better to save where you can. No one knows how long the journey will be; pace yourself and allow the Universe to help you through these lovely organisations. These are people waiting to give you God's love through them to make your prayers come true. Be open, and allow for the love to flow to you.

Are prescriptions included or not?

Many health insurance companies include prescription medicines in the coverage, which is a huge blessing because those are medicines one has to take as part of the treatment. These include diabetic meds, chemo pills, insulin, pancreatic enzyme pills, seizure meds, epileptic pens, and the list goes on. One may think, oh, it's ok; in most countries like India and Pakistan, medicine is so reasonably priced that it still doesn't make sense to buy health insurance and waste so much money. But do you know that Creon pills (pancreatic enzyme pills) cost in the hundreds of dollars each month, Ozempic (diabetic injection) costs from 200-500 dollars a month, arthritis injections can cost up to a thousand dollars a month and chemo pills, of course, are exceptionally expensive also.

Which insurance?

There are many different insurance companies out there with different plans. It is extremely important to do your research and find the one that suits your needs and/or your family's needs. There are many things to consider:

1) Single or family plan?

2) In-patient and/or Out-patient coverage?

3) Deductible or no deductible?

4) Which country coverage?

    a) Just your country of residence

    b) International excluding the United States

    c) International including the United States

    d) If you live in a country that does not have good healthcare, you may need to have a Helivac option?

    e) If you have problems and possible violence in your country, then you need an expatriation/evacuation option also.

5) Sometimes, they cover prescription meds, also

6) Monthly or yearly payments?

7) Dental or no dental?

8) How long before pregnancy does one need to buy health

insurance for mom and baby in case something goes wrong? It can be extremely costly if there is a problem with the baby: incubator, tests, possible surgeries or procedures.

9) Direct billing or pay and claim?

10) Which hospitals does it cover in your country?

11) Do they cover pre-existing conditions?

    a) If not, then how long do they need you to pay before they cover it, 1 or 2 years for some insurance companies?

    b) Most do not cover pre-existing conditions, or they charge a huge premium.

    c) Read carefully everything about pre-existing conditions; they may also exclude related conditions from coverage.

12) Will you be dealing with the insurance company directly?

    a) Agents can be extremely annoying. You think they will fight for you, but they can become more painful to deal with than directly dealing with the insurance company. But they can be extremely helpful too so keep good relations with them.

    b) Management companies can also be nice or mean depending. The problem with management companies is that they may change often and then the policy can change which will leave you stranded especially if you need a year or 2 of pre-existing conditions to follow.

    c) It is best to buy insurance through the agents, but when going through illness, it's sometimes best to deal with the insurance company representatives directly. They are more compassionate since they deal directly with patients and their families on a daily basis. Their empathy makes them understand you better and allow for things the management and agents may not.

13) It might be cheaper to make a group for the health insurance as the premium will be lower per person.

How to put a claim

If you are getting a planned surgery and the hospital is covered under your insurance, then the hospital will take care of the claim, provided there is a direct payment agreement with that hospital. If they have a 'pay and claim' relationship, then that means you pay and claim later with a claim form filled out by the doctor. In this case, you will send the signed form by the doctor to the insurance company yourself. They will have to approve it after the treatment is done, so you won't know till they decide if they are covering it or not. Then there is a whole long wait time for the money to get processed and reach your account again. Good luck with the 'pay and claim' option. It can be painful. Although many insurance companies have become well digitised with apps that make life easier and more efficient.

Important: When there is an emergency, and you take the patient to the emergency unit, please call the insurance company right away, or if you have an app, then fill in the required form. This will ensure that the insurance company is alerted and can start the process in case the patient needs further care, as they usually only cover emergency care after the patient has been in a bed at the hospital for more than a certain amount of hours for in-patient coverage. For example, if the patient is there and is released from the emergency unit (not counting the waiting room time) before the minimum required hours, then the visit will not be covered by the insurance unless you have out-patient coverage as well.

Direct or pay and claim

It is imperative that you check if the hospital has a direct payment or a 'pay and claim' agreement with the insurance company. Direct payment does not require you to use any of your money, nor does it ask for a guarantee. For 'pay and claim' options, they require a guarantee for which they will block more than necessary amounts and may add more as the treatments go on. The sad thing is that the money goes quickly, but once the insurance company accepts the claim, it takes forever to return the money. Moreover, when it comes time for you to claim the money, they can come up with ridiculous reasons not to pay, and then you may have to fight to get your money back.

Fighting insurance

Emergency or regular in-patient claims or out-patient claims - please read every little detail of your insurance booklet from top to bottom. As with every other insurance coverage, health coverage will try to pay the bare minimum possible, and they will fight to save their money where they can. Just like any other business, when it comes to taking money, they are all sweet and in a hurry, but when it comes time to pay the money, they are slow and feisty if need be. The craziest experience I had with the insurance company was when my dad got diagnosed with COPD (Chronic Obstructive Pulmonary Disorder) during Covid time (Jan 2020). Some crazy doctor of his had put in the hospital notes that in 2009, 'maybe' my dad had asthma, even though no test had shown this and nor was my dad taking any ongoing asthma medication. Unfortunately, he needed to be hospitalised in January 2021 for pneumonia-type symptoms, and because the insurance companies had been exasperated with claims, they gave me a big battle to cover my dad's illness based on that doctor's notes. He needed to use a bi-pap machine at home, and we kept a nurse, but these were out-patient expenses, and he only had in-patient coverage, so these were on us. The hospital charges, which the insurance always covered without question, were under debate with the insurance company.

The management of the health insurance company had just changed recently, so I didn't have an ally in the representatives. I had to rely on the agent we had bought the insurance from to fight my fight, but he was biased and took their side. My dad passed away in his sleep in March of 2021. The insurance was fighting coverage of his hospital stay even after his death. Can you believe it? At the start of my grieving process, with my dad gone in the blink of an eye, these horrible human beings were hell-bent on arguing with me. I just told them, "What kind of human beings are you? Instead of offering me condolences and having empathy, you are telling me that my dead father's bill needs to be paid and hounding me with arguments about how you cannot cover it. I don't have the brain space to think of all this right now, so please just charge me since you are so insensitive and greedy." I had already given them all the proof I had of him not ever having asthma; therefore, the pre-existing condition wasn't there for them to disregard the COPD bills. I just didn't have any more energy to fight them. They ended up feeling really bad after that and paid the bills.

The key to optimum insurance coverage is to get to know a representative and stick to them for the whole case. This will make your life easier as the person knows the case as you go along and will feel the process with you, which will lead to complying with you when needs be rather than the company. In my mom's time, the management was consistent, and I made a few friends in the insurance claim department. They even asked me to give my testimonial for their website. One of them even came to meet me when I was visiting the country where they were located.

Insurance companies will always fight to pay the least amount possible or not pay at all if you don't stay on top of things. You have to be assertive, not aggressive, but rather firm and stern. Then only will they take you seriously. Try to keep all documentation with the dates, times, and names of agents for future rebuttals since they can come up with arguments at any time. This is especially certain when they change their management, and therefore, the conditions may change. Even after the patient's death, I would say to keep the documents for a bit longer until all claims and cases are closed. Some hospitals have delayed billing, so you may get bills for a bit longer than you would anticipate.

Hospitals have special discounts for Private Payment.

Please, please, please! For those of you without insurance, do ask for a discount. Hospitals charge insurance companies way too much, so they usually have leeway to give discounts to people paying privately. Yes! Fortunately, the hospital accounting department does have a heart sometimes, so take advantage of it. It's there for a reason. Even they understand how Over the Top the bills can amount to at the end of complicated diseases. It's tough for even the richest people to lose big amounts of money. At the end of the day, none of us like to lose even small amounts of money for nothing. So forget your shame and ask away!! You may be happily surprised!

CHAPTER 7

SELF-HELP FOR CAREGIVER:

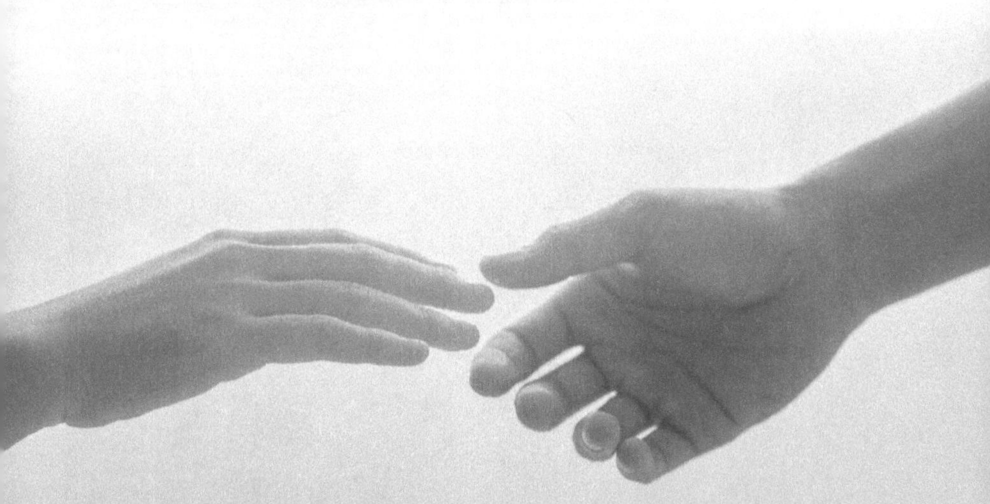

P**hysical, mental, emotional, and spiritual effects**

They say everything in life is a choice. I used to wonder how a person getting sick could be a choice. How can a girl of age 9 getting raped in the middle of a village be a choice? I think I finally understand. The action itself is not the choice. The choice is in what we make of the experience the action provides for us.

My mom getting sick was not her choice. I don't think anyone in their right mind chooses to die a slow and painful death. The choice is in what we do with the time we have together in the middle of all the pain and craziness. We can fight with each other and be depressed, or we can choose to be happy with each other and enjoy whatever time we have together when the ill parent has energy. Today, it is my choice: either I learn from the experiences I had with my parents, or I can sit here and cry about why God did this to me, and everyone else has a family of their own and I don't. There is so much to learn from my experiences, why would I cry to God? Not having anyone to love has helped me love God directly. While I loved my parents or loved another human being, they became the idea of God I prayed to, which is so wrong. Maybe God loved me so much that He took away everyone that came between me and Him so I could learn to love Him directly and have that beautiful one-on-one relationship with Him. I learned to talk to

Him about my fears and complaints. Like a sieve, everyone around me who was not aligned with me spiritually slipped through the holes and became estranged. Only my spiritual tribe, attracted to me along the way, remained.

I am so grateful to God that He afforded me awareness during my mom's illness, leading me to the choice of changing myself in order to revamp my relationship with her. Why would anyone want to fight with someone who is not well? I think it's cowardice at its height. When people are strong, yes, by all means, argue and stand up for yourselves. But when the other person is at his/her weakest, why would you pick a fight with them? Only cowards or bullies can do that. Take the higher ground, be the better person, and start the journey to mend all your differences. Time is running out. The illness is a wake-up call, not just for the ill person, but for everyone around. Wake up before it is too late.

Even while writing this book, I remember asking my mom, "Who will keep this family together after you go?" She turned around and said, "You will keep them together." At that point, that was the most unrealistic thought to cross anyone's mind! Haha, I was always the black sheep of the family. Nobody, and I mean nobody, in the family listened to anything I had to say, so I am sure she told each one of us the same thing. She was right though, we definitely kept it together as a team! Thank God!

Her vote of confidence, approval of my life, and belief in me are what got me through my tough days. I am so unbelievably grateful to God that He gave me the chance to make amends with her before she left this world. I would never be able to live with myself if we had not fixed our relationship. Furthermore, to live without feeling unconditional love leads to many psychological and emotional issues. One of these issues affected my personal life deeply: I didn't know what love was because I didn't feel it from anyone in my life. How do you recognise something you have never felt? How do you feel a feeling that you have never felt?

After my mom passed, I automatically switched to being there for my dad. My dad didn't think I would be there, although he was closest to me before my mom got sick. Somehow, while my mom was sick, he thought I would not be there for him, but he was still my dad, and I loved him to death. It's weird because all my life, he was the one who was 'my person' in the family to the point where I would pray to God to take me before him because I didn't want to live in a world without him. Unfortunately, God didn't listen to my prayer.

I was 40 and single when my mom got sick. Before they die, every parent in Southeast Asia would like to see each of their children settled with a husband or wife. One brother and I were still single at the time. By the time my mom passed away, I had just turned 43. Now, you have to understand that it is old in my culture not to be married. Plus, my biological clock was ticking alarm bells as a last call to have children of my own. My mom, on the other hand, just before she passed away, told me: "You are fine on your own. I know you will be okay." She used to call me her 'son' as a compliment, haha. I don't know if being a 'son' is a compliment, but I know she was trying to say that, in her eyes, I could do whatever I put my mind to. She was trying to praise me because she saw that I could drive, organise anything they needed, cook, clean, arrange appointments, talk to the doctors, clean her wounds, fight with whoever I needed to, reach out to anybody we needed like lawyers and immigration personnel, and above all I could protect her from anyone who tried to make her lose hope. She knew she was safe with me and that I would do whatever I could to keep her fighting in comfort.

Losing whose life?

Whose life are we losing, really? The patient is sick, yes, but aren't you losing your life too? It may not seem like it at the moment. You may feel you are taking the 'higher' ground, and you feel all 'Mother Theresa'-ish or Edhi-esque, but those are the paths they have chosen, and that is their life's work. You had a life before this. You will need to have a life after this. How long this is going to go on for, nobody knows. Are you okay with forgoing 5 years, 10 years, 15 years, or more of your life, your youth? Are you okay with having regrets about not doing that course, giving up that job/promotion, not having babies, not getting married, not attending your niece's wedding or not being accepted in society anymore because you cannot relate to people at their superficial level anymore because your life is so heavy and serious?

Exercise:

When we are taking care of a patient, everyone focuses on the patient, including the caregiver. No one thinks about the caregiver, not even the caregiver him/herself. Just like on the plane, when the oxygen masks come down, they tell us to wear ours first and then help other people or our own children. We are no good to anyone else if we don't look after ourselves first. For example, if while taking care of the patient, the caregiver gets sick and ends up in bed or in the hospital, then who will take care of the patient? Or, if the caregiver has a mental breakdown, he or she will not be able to handle the responsibilities required of them as the caregiver. Therefore, taking care of one's health, both physical and mental, is very important as a caregiver.

The first element of taking care of oneself would be to make sure you are physically healthy while taking care of your loved one. Exercising is the most important way to keep yourself physically fit. Even 30 minutes to an hour a day of walking in nature or on the treadmill will keep your body and mind healthy. Another option could be to take an exercise class in a gym or club nearby. If that is not an easy-to-do option, then there are many exercises one can find online to do at home for free.

Options for exercising:

1) Walk or run outside

2) Go up and down stairs

3) Yoga poses

4) Stretching on mat

5) Biking

6) Play a sport

7) Gym (ex, treadmill, strength training, boxing)

8) Exercise class online or in-person (ex: aerobic, belly-dancing, Zumba, pilates)

Another way to take care of yourself physically is to monitor your food intake and timing. One either ends up not eating or eating too much. We end up munching on random things while waiting at the appointments or while running around. The patient's food is monitored closely and given extra attention, but the caregiver's meals are not planned. Also, the caregiver is so busy running around and making sure everything is okay with the patient that most of the time, they eat in a hurry or grab what is around. This way, the caregiver ends up being undernourished by skipping meals or eating small portions. On the other hand, the caregiver can be over nourished by eating unhealthy food like fast food or chocolates, etc, causing weight gain. Once we put on weight, it's a vicious cycle. We start wearing comfortable clothing with elastic waistbands, and before we know it, our weight is out of control. This causes insecurity, which makes you want to be more shabby and sedentary, which will inevitably cause diseases like diabetes and high blood pressure.

Passion and Hobbies

Although it sounds crazy, this is the time to indulge in the activities you enjoy the most, especially if you are not working at the time or even if you are. A little bit of time out for yourself is essential for the mental, physical and emotional peace of the carer. You are vital to the recovery of the patient, so you must take care of yourself. When we take a little time out for ourselves, we come back happier and refueled. We are better people to be around for the patient, and we see things around us in a better light. We will get less frustrated, and we may even be able to be light-hearted and jovial with the patient.

Examples of activities include:

1) Painting

2) Art therapy

3) Music therapy

4) Horse-riding

5) Racquet sports or other sports

6) Scrapbooking

7) Dancing

8) Walking

9) Hiking, and so on

Outlet/entertainment

Once you aren't happy with yourself, you tend to stay home and give up socialising. It is imperative to go out and take time for your enjoyment. Don't abandon yourself. Self-care includes taking care of your mental and emotional health too. Make sure you go to movies, spend time with friends, watch your favourite shows, create 'me' time and log these into your schedule. Socialising and getting love have proven benefits to one's health. If you replenish the love and energy within you, then only can you pass that on to the patient.

There are many online games available also: Sudoku, Words with Friends, Scrabble, Candy Crush, etc. All these come in handy when you are waiting in the waiting room for a doctor's appointment for both you and the patient. They help keep the mind deterred and occupied. Sometimes, all we need is a bit of a distraction and not a fully focused commitment to an activity, as we will need to snap back to real life in a jiffy. Portable games and activities that are doable in spurts are a perfect distraction!

We are lucky if someone thinks of us and offers us a coffee with which to put our feet up and watch a movie after a long day of taking care of the patient. But why depend on luck? Make yourself lucky and take time out for that coffee and a movie. You deserve it. After long hours of taking care of other people, your body gets depleted of energy. It needs refuelling, so don't ignore it. If no one else will provide you with the love and care you need to replenish your energy, don't ignore yourself. You will burn out and crash if you keep going like that. Even one hour of sitting with a coffee and doing nothing or walking or watching a comedy show, etc, will give you so much happiness and respite. This way, you can go back to being the carer with a happier mind and more love for the patient. You will be a better person for yourself, for them, and for everybody else around you.

On the other hand, if you keep ignoring and abandoning yourself, you will lose yourself. You will burn out and crash. Once you lose yourself, you are no good to yourself or others. To maximise everyone's care, you have to take care of yourself first and foremost!

Researching patient care:

When we first find out our loved one has a terminal illness, our brains freeze, and we are in utter shock. The mind doesn't work, and generally, we have no clue where to begin. Please, please, please, do not start googling statistics of illness! Keep positive and hopeful, and do your best. The patient will feed off your energy and your mindset. The day you give up hope or are negative, they will also give up!

If there is anything you need to research, it's these:

1) Appointments

2) Insurance Coverage: In-patient only or both in-patient and out-patient

3) Financials: to cover everything (it's going to be expensive!)

4) Hygiene and health of the patient

5) Nutrition: Food and supplements

6) Driving if distant or flying to a better care area

7) Rights of the patient in and out of the hospital

8) Alternate treatments

9) Clinical trials

10) Meditation and spiritual guidance - prayers and meditations

11) Therapies

12) Most importantly: Loved ones should be notified and make a schedule for visits/calls.

Research help

Above all, do not be scared to ask for help. We all feel the need to do everything alone, but you will burn out. So, make sure you delegate duties and distribute the responsibilities to alleviate stress.

Stress is a huge player at this point. We don't realise but we are stressed about the patient but we also get stressed in being responsible for everything that needs to be done. So take the help when offered. This is not the time to be holier than thou or superheroes. Grace is of utmost benefit - gracefully accept that you are only human and you will be a happier and less frustrated human being with a bit of extra help from others.

Boundaries

This leads us to the concept of 'boundaries'. We were all brought up to not be 'selfish' and to sacrifice for the other. Empathy and compassion were idealised, and we were forced to give up our needs and wants for the betterment of others, especially family or loved ones. As perfect as this sounds, it is not healthy at all. If you are depleted of energy and become frustrated, you are of no use to the patient or anybody around you. You will add strain to your relationships with the patient and everyone else. All your efforts will go to waste as this behaviour will negate everything you have done so far. This is why boundaries are a MUST!!! You have to learn to listen to your body and say 'NO' when you can't do something or realise that you need your alone time or whatever else you need. Respect yourself, and then only will others respect you. People-pleasing doesn't work because, inevitably, someone will have an issue with you. As the adage goes: "We can please some of the people some of the time, or we can please some of the people all of the time, but we cannot please all of the people all of the time or even some of the time." Nice-ness is not sustainable; goodness is. Yes, for the overall good of the situation, push yourself, but don't force yourself to be nice just to please others to your own detriment. It serves no one because when you get fed up, you will regret it.

Pace your energy

It's better to pace yourself. No one knows how long the patient will take to get better or if it will be a lifelong treatment. Neglecting yourself will create a snowball effect of tiredness and frustration which will come out in the craziest ways. It's better to keep your physical, mental and emotional health balanced throughout by keeping your days balanced and healthy.

Burnout is the inevitable result of the carer caring for everyone but themselves. If you reach the point of burnout, the patient will be left uncared for, and you will not be able to take care of them or yourself. We don't want to reach this point. It starts with frustration, getting irritated at the patient and others around for little things. We feel like we need to control everything, and everything has to be done a certain way - our way! But it needn't be that way. Others can do things in different ways with love, and it's okay. Different ways don't equate to wrong ways. They are just different, and variety is the spice of life. The patient may just appreciate the change, and also, being the main carer, they kind of get sick of you (pun intended!) just like you get sick of them. It's the taking-for-granted syndrome that whoever we care about, we are the toughest on them. Take your space, and give them their space. They need a bit of independence, and others need to give their love and attention to the patient and also give them all their space. If there is an emergency or something important, trust me, they will call you!

Keep your autonomy

Another key point is to keep your life map intact. Know your purpose in life other than intertwining with the patient's purpose. Make sure you don't give up on your life and your priorities. Maybe you can't keep your 9-5 job, but you can find a way to stay up to date in the field so that you can come back to it at a later date without losing too much in the process. One of the worst things is to have nothing to come back to after losing a loved one. Life has revolved too long around the patient, and we are used to getting attention because of them and having a full and busy life. Unfortunately, after they pass on, that attention and fullness of life goes away in a minute. You are left alone with an emptiness in your life that is impossible to comprehend. The immense grief one goes through is so confusing, and the pain is multiplied by the silence and lack one feels without the dependency on the patient and their life.

Hold on to what you have! Yes, shocking, isn't it? It's not just the patient who is dependent on you; you become dependent on the patient, too. We need to hold on to something that's "yours". For example, work, relationships, hobbies, etc.; otherwise, you become the shadow of the patient and lose your identity. Everything becomes associated with the patient's needs, wants and health requirements. This identity crisis will come to haunt you after, god forbid, something happens to the patient. Keep your autonomy and identity, or it will take a long time for you to get them back.

Yes, we change a lot during this time, but one shouldn't lose the base of their personality. Don't get pushed over by people. Don't let them take advantage of you. Don't let yourself take advantage of your capabilities, and don't stretch yourself so much that you break.

Find people in the same situation to share experiences and feel 'normal'

Hey, you aren't alone in this…we are all going through the same thing, or if not already going through it, we have been or will be soon! Find a support group or find people in a similar situation and share your ideas and concerns: Misery loves company. It's sad but true. Knowing that others are going through whatever problems we have makes it so much easier to bear through the experience. Funnily enough, you may even be able to laugh at some of the things you are going through when you start opening up to other people taking care of their parents. A lot of experiences feel personal and hurtful until we realise that every parent-child relationship has those same frustrations and issues. Don't fret! Most of the time, love gets hidden behind the most awful expressions and actions. We just have to stay aware and have an open heart to see the good parts.

Under these circumstances, socialising with your regular people might become a bit difficult. After spending all your time at hospitals and around patients, your whole being is used to illness, death and dying. Therefore, it becomes very difficult to socialise and interact with the same people we used to. Conversations we used to indulge in will begin to seem trivial since our priorities have become different. This is why one needs to find a new tribe. The kind of tribe that relates to your new stage in life with common experiences.

Dealing with Stress

Stress is the root cause of most illnesses. It can cause a 'flight or flight' response in our system; it causes emotional eating in some people, it can tighten the body, and it can cause veins to constrict. All these result in a person getting diabetes, blood pressure issues, cardiovascular issues and all kinds of other health issues with the added weight. We must balance stress with exercise. There is a famous analogy one makes with animals: just as an animal shakes itself to release stress, humans need to shake and move their bodies to remove their stress, too. Activities to engage in to help relieve stress can be racquet sports, horse riding, Zumba classes, aerobic exercises, belly dancing, sky-diving, running, walking, etc. Whatever you want, just do something! Other non-physical ways to de-stress can include: reading, journaling, spending time in nature, being still, connecting with like-minded and supportive friends, or even a short stay-cation.

CHAPTER 8

SPIRITUAL DIMENSION

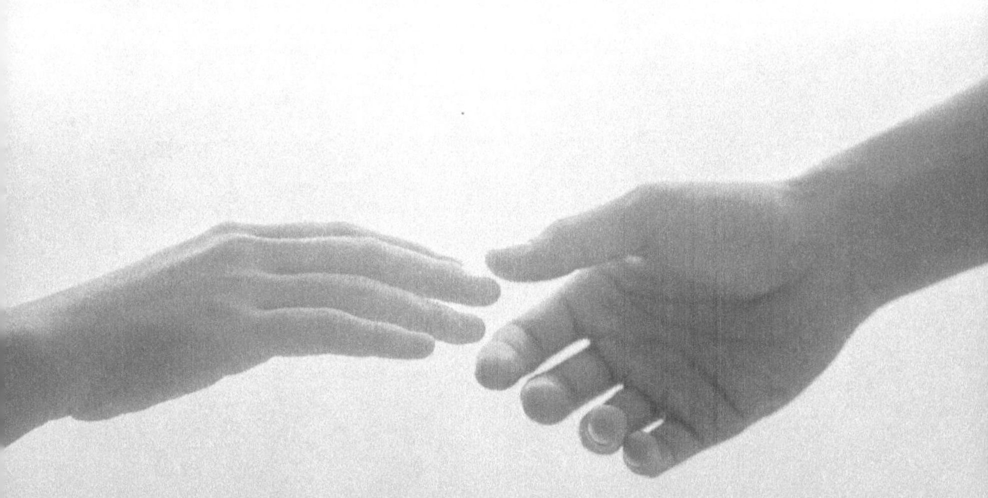

Prayers for the patient

If the patient is religious or spiritual, their faith helps to give them solace and peace regarding their illness. It helps them surrender the fate of the disease to something beyond themselves and the doctors. Also, it allows for hope that things will get better and their lives will go back to a sort of 'normal' eventually. Surrendering and having hope are two things that really help to keep one's mind at ease. This can possibly prevent the patient from blaming or getting upset at doctors if the treatment doesn't have the desired outcome. Also, it keeps the patient from getting frustrated and angry, protecting the people around them from their wrath when they vent.

1) Faith-related prayers

2) Guided or Unguided Meditation

3) Mantras

4) Positive affirmations

Another point where faith-related guidance becomes important is if, unfortunately, the treatment doesn't work and the patient has to think about leaving this world. Most hospitals will call in a faith representative according to the patient's beliefs. These people of God or spiritual guides will prepare the patient for the difficult time of death and its implications. For people who believe in an afterlife with death being a reunion with the most loved one, God, it is important to feel happy at the reunion versus the concept of leaving loved ones in this world.

As advanced as we are, dealing with the death of a loved one is still terribly complicated. Our definition of life is intertwined with our relationships, and we get so used to having certain people around that we don't know how to live without them. That doesn't mean we can't, it just takes time to relearn how to live life in this novel capacity. The world can be scary, but it has some wonderful people in it. You just need time and effort to find the right people to help you get through this most difficult time in your life. I promise you: the person and their memories will always be with you, but the pain will get less as the days go by. You will learn to live and be happy again. Don't feel guilty. They want you to be happy living your life.

Prayers to keep the sanity of everyone around

The carer and loved ones of the patient will have a lot of pressure and responsibility, which may cause anxiety and panic attacks just as the patient might have. The unknown tends to have this impact on us, and having a religion or some kind of faith or spirituality to turn to really helps. It is superb in keeping us rooted in life and providing us with a sense of security. The idea of fate and destiny provides an excuse to blame someone other than ourselves, and there is no repercussion for it; rather, it is required by the nature of religion and the Higher Power. When one has a strong grasp on these ideologies, it provides a sense of relief and calm in these most highly stressful and painful situations.

Grounding tools

You must keep a routine. Chances are you have left your job to take care of your loved one, but that doesn't mean you have abandoned your life. Meet your friends, exercise, read and above all, continue your faith-based activities. These will all keep you rooted and will give you energy, which will fuel you with energy to give to the patient. Continuing with your work and activities as much as you can will offer a semblance of 'normality' and allow you the psychological stability to handle the situation better.

Other physically grounding tools include:

1) Walking on grass, on the beach, or in nature.

2) Epsom salt baths provide rejuvenation and relaxation.

3) Calming and soothing activities include:

a) Meditating

b) Partaking in faith groups.

4) Physical touch

a) Hugs

b) Massages

5) Being still

Spiritual Impact

Spirituality, believing in a Higher Power above us, is very important to me. I know not everyone believes in this. I grew up in a semi-religious home with a secular worldview, but we were taught never to discuss religion. Religion was understood to be a personal matter, and everyone may have one, but it was no one else's business. It was only important to view a person as 'good' or 'not so good' as a human being. My parents taught us to respect all religions as we grew up in the Democratic Republic of Congo. My parents were born there, and so were three of us siblings, and we all grew up there. Our lineage goes to India, and our relatives lived in Pakistan and Canada while growing up. We travelled all over every year while growing up, and now the five of us siblings are spread over 4 continents.

In my first year of university, I took Philosophy 101, in which the whole year centred around the question: Does God exist? It was a crucial point in the evolution of my religious-spiritual growth. I wanted to challenge myself to see if I just believed in God for the heck of it or if my faith was really truly mine. I realised during that course we may never be able to prove the existence of God on paper, but life and its experiences show us His might, and He lets us feel Him if we are open to it. At least for me, it felt like that. I came out of that course feeling extremely strong and sure in my conviction that there is a Higher power above us holding this world together and guiding us through life.

From then onwards, I started seeing the coincidences and 'the invisible hand of God' in all things. Even though I didn't follow my religion traditionally, nor did I practise any of the rituals, the foundation was fortified, providing me with a firm starting point. Most people believe in their religions so strongly while trying to make sense of it from within that bubble. I erased everything, started from scratch, and started thinking from without. It was easy for me because I was from a country that never allowed me to call myself from there owing to the colour of my skin. I was from nowhere, yet from everywhere. The countries I resembled the people of were fighting each other, and I didn't fit in because I didn't speak or dress like them; I only ate like them. I studied in an American School and Canadian University and eventually got the nationality, but I am definitely not American or Canadian from any angle whatsoever except for the way I speak and dress. I had a British passport at one point, but there is absolutely no English side to me. I spent more time in Belgium and Switzerland than in the UK, being from a Belgian colony and from the French-speaking world. Since I literally am from nowhere and have no loyalty to any country but love all of them for different reasons, it was easy to break down my religious and spiritual thinking to the common denominator = God, Allah, Bhagwan, universe, higher power, nature, etc (whatever you want to call it!). Reaching this ground zero (or rather the highest point, depends how one sees it), this point was an aha moment for me, and nothing from then on could shatter my faith. My belief in God was indelibly marked in my heart and soul.

So the day my mom collapsed, and we knew this was something serious, I made a promise to God with my decision to be her primary caregiver for as long as needed. While I was caring for her, this soul connection made me do things I never before imagined I could do. I had enough energy for ten people. I had never cooked before in my life, yet I was cooking all three meals fresh every day. I was her secretary, the driver, the cook, the carer, her nurse and whatever else was needed. My days were non-stop from morning till night. The difference between pre and post-me was so stark that my brother even commented once: 'You are like a robot; how are you doing all this?' Honestly, I don't even know. There was some force beyond me. I had no idea about cancers and illnesses in general before that, but somehow, as soon as we went into an appointment, I would understand the doctors, who would talk to me somehow, knowing 'she is the one to talk to'. I give all the credit to God because, before every appointment and every morning when I woke up, I closed my eyes and saw the light of His being enveloping me and connecting with the light inside me. I would then pray for Him to stay with me and work His magic through my being. I started this journey by telling Him that I knew this was the right thing for me to do in His eyes, so I would do it to please Him. I truly believed He listened to me and was with me every step of the way through my journey as a carer for my mother and father.

Whenever anything good or bad happens, if we believe God is good, then we must believe that everything He makes happen in this world to us and around us has to be good, too. There is a method to the madness (metaphorically) He creates around us. We must believe whatever is happening is because of Allah or God's will, and therefore, it is for our betterment. Maybe there is a lesson for us to learn, or it could be a lesson others need to learn from us. Sometimes, it is easier in hindsight to see why things happened the way they did. When we see the lessons we learnt, we may even be grateful for the hardships we went through.

Having faith is a great way to keep your peace and sanity. After my mom passed away, my dad and our siblings were grieving, but everyone kept strong in front of each other. I didn't know how to balance the grief while pretending to be strong living with my dad. I was in a predicament, so I decided to get therapy from a psychoanalyst who had done some great work on my friend - I loved the changes in my friend. I took therapy sessions for over a year, three times a week. He became a really good friend, haha, which goes without saying. At the end of the year, or maybe over a year, I had learned everything I could from him (and spent way too much money!). I then decided that therapy is great for helping you deal with real-life situations and for helping you think like the other people around you to create harmony. But peace of mind can only come with a peaceful heart and soul, which in turn can only come from the belief in a spiritual entity to whom we can submit fully and trust wholeheartedly. Until I didn't incorporate discipline in my connection with God through meditation or rituals, the anxiety wouldn't stop, and the calm that I had during my mom's illness eluded me. I just couldn't get the feeling back.

After my dad passed away, the anxiety snowballed. I felt like the rug was pulled out from under my feet. My whole existence had revolved around my parents. They were the centre of my world, the core of my existence. I had always prayed to God to take me before my parents. I even prayed for Him to give me my mom's illness instead of her and let her live longer. I didn't see the point of me being here when I had no dependents or obligations. They had so much more to give to this world and were so much more needed. I could never understand why God took away the people I loved and kept me here. These thoughts bothered me a lot after my dad passed away. I didn't understand how I was supposed to go on without them. Even though I was the rebel in the family, the black sheep who lived far away from them for most of my life, I never cut the cord. There was an indelible cord connecting me with them. I could not define my life without them. They were my everything, and the world just didn't make sense without them.

Many of us get peeved off by the inundation of people after a death and feel harassed by the rituals and commotion. When it happens, be grateful for them. They are a source of comfort and care. The rituals set you in motion, providing you with discipline in connecting with God, which will ease your pain and relieve you of your loneliness and sadness. He is the one who encompasses you in His unconditional and ever-providing love. We seek groundedness, and the higher power is the only one that can give us that consistently and permanently. Everything else is temporary. People will leave you, or they will die. He is the only one who will be there, always.

Little miracles

In the time after death, you will see many coincidences and if you are aware and open, you will see the hand of God in everything that happens. Losing a loved one puts us in a zone that is highly spiritual. We are on a different plane of existence. They say that our loved ones come back to us in other forms, namely animals and insects. The most commonly believed object to represent the dead is the white butterfly. After my brother-in-law passed away, his children received tremendous comfort in seeing the rare sight of white butterflies in their backyard and in the cemetery.

The little miracles of life are what make us happy and intact, both mentally and emotionally. When those two parts of us are taken care of, the physical tends to stay balanced. Yes, we all want to see our loved ones recover fully and continue their lives as normal. Sometimes, this is not possible, but it is not for us to foresee or control. Therefore, the best thing to do is to focus on small accomplishments and victories. When we celebrate along the journey, it gets easier to accept the situation and to normalise it. For example, if the patient has been vomiting and can now eat without regurgitating anything, that is a serious win! If the patient has been getting infections and is in and out of the hospital and all of a sudden, they get cured of the infection, but they still have fourth-stage cancer, they still won the infection.

Celebrating each win will give the patient the fight they need to tackle the next challenge, and it will also give them a reason to appreciate where they are. If they feel gratitude for each step, it will boost their morale and encourage them to keep going. Small steps are easier to face than the whole mountain all at once.

Gratitude

Gratitude is everything. When we are grateful, our energy levels rise, and our energy field becomes bigger and wider. Gratefulness makes the law of attraction kick in in a positive way. The higher our energies are, the higher the levels of life events we attract, of which love is the highest. Love and gratitude will increase our potential to have an abundant life in every aspect. If you, as a carer, can carry gratitude and high levels of energy to induce abundance, then imagine how that would impact your patient. You will heighten their energy and add to their levels to attract the highest abundance of all kinds, including the restoration of health.

Connection between patient and carer

There is a very deep connection between the carer and patient that will inevitably cause them to be in tune with each other's needs and feelings to the point where the carer may even be able to sense the physical and emotional state of the patient. The carer will have to be the cheerleader for the patient and keep the patient positive and hopeful. It may even come to the point where if the carer loses hope, the patient will sense this and give up hope, too. This may seem heavy and extreme, but it is a very real connection that forms.

The dependency of the patient on the carer is such that when the carer is away, the patient may even fall physically ill just because they are used to believing they are well because of the carer. The opposite becomes true too: the carer starts believing that if they aren't there or if they miss a beat, the patient will suffer because of them.

Fears and Regrets

In certain cases we can start blaming ourselves and having regrets. Our fears cause our brains to go into panic mode and we start second-guessing our decisions as we get filled with regrets either pointing fingers at others or then being self-critical and putting ourselves down. There are a few key points to remember when we get hard on ourselves if anything goes wrong.

1) It is imperative that we stop criticising ourselves and second-guessing our decisions. What is going to happen is going to happen. We need to give it our best and make the best decisions under the circumstances.

2) Secondly, try to stop criticising others and judging each other. In such situations, we all get very stressed since we care so much about the well-being of our loved ones. When things go wrong, it's very easy to point fingers at others or, worse yet, at ourselves. Try to keep in mind that everybody is doing their best, and that's all anyone can do. If things go wrong, it's not anyone's fault. Some things are meant to be the way they are for bigger reasons we may not ever comprehend.

3) The only way to prevent all of the above from happening, is firstly, stop all fear. This fear ends up terrorising your being. It keeps you in fight or flight mode tensing up your body causing all kinds of issues. These issues can lead to more complicated diseases and illnesses in the future if you don't address them in due time.

4) To begin with, if you are kind and compassionate to yourself, you may prevent all issues and create a beautiful, calm environment for the patient and for everyone around. I am sure you are saying it's not me who is sick; it's the patient. Why do I need to be so extra to myself? Why not? Why can't we be as nice to ourselves as we are to the patient? Why do we, as human beings, always put ourselves last and forget to take care of ourselves? If you find it difficult to do this, make a list of your fears and give them to God. You must believe that He will do the best that can be done. Whatever happens is in His hands, and He knows how much you can handle and your limits. He knows best for the patient, too, and He has a plan. As they say, We plan, and God executes better than we can imagine. He watches out for everyone to create the best fate for each.

5) For both you and the patient, try to keep away from negativity. This reminds me of a time when my uncle in Toronto became comatose in the hospital. "According to the University of California, Santa Barbara's UCSB Sciencline website, the brain can withstand three to six minutes without oxygen before brain damage occurs." (www.spinalcord.com/blog/what-happens-to-the-brain-after-a-lack-of-oxygen#)   My uncle was alone in the hospital room, so no one knows how long it had been since he had collapsed before the doctor and nurses tried to resuscitate him. They kept going for over 20 minutes before they got him back. The doctor then put ice all over his body in order to slow down the brain's need for oxygen, and once he was 'chilled, ' they slowly brought his body temperature up to our regular temperature. When she started allowing people to see him, she first gave us a

pep talk: "I do not work in the ICU to have my patients pass away. I fight hard to keep my patients alive. Whoever wants to cross this line into the ICU unit has to come with a positive frame of mind, namely, that my patient is going to fight and survive this condition. I do not allow any negativity in my ICU unit. If you don't think like this, please don't enter." My uncle recovered within a few days with his mental faculties intact. This is the mindset one should have while caregiving. It's the only way to keep everyone's spirits lifted and full of hope.

DEALING WITH GRIEF

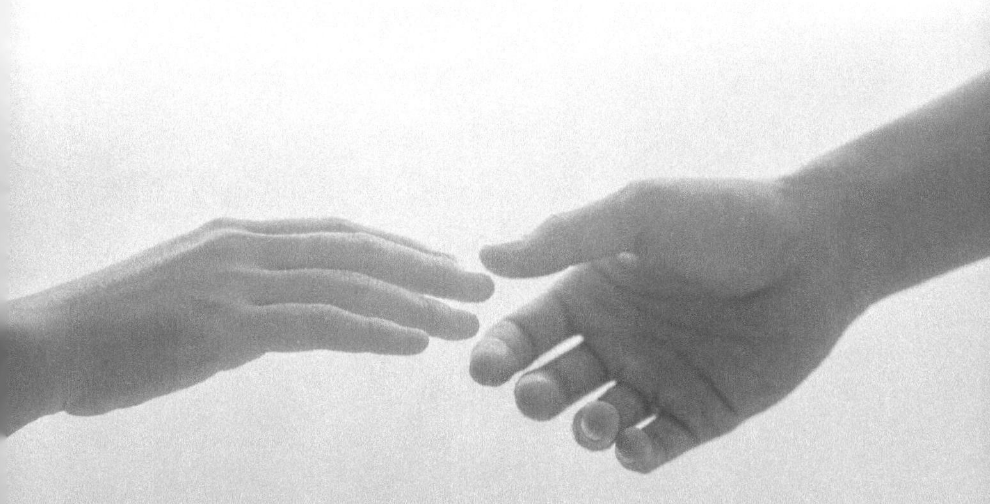

Dealing with the loss of a person from life

Grief comes to everyone at one time or another. There is no preparation for grief. The first time we lose a loved one who we interact with every day of our lives, the one who is happy and sad for us, the one who is the most emotionally attached to us, it can be devastating. The finality of death doesn't resemble anything else one can ever go through in life. It's not temporary. We can never see them again, speak to them again or hug them. It's not like they went on a vacation and will come back someday. They are gone forever, never to return. You can never hear their voice another time, you can never hug them or smell them. You cannot call them and get advice or run to them for attention and love. It is a permanent loss; as permanent as it gets. It takes time to reach this point, but when the permanence of their absence dawns on you, this is when you truly start processing your grief. It is a journey. We all mistakenly think we will be over it after a few months or a year. You will go through many different steps until you accept the loss, carrying the grief around with you, receding into the background of everything else. Even though the pain stays forever, it will get better, I promise - just be patient and let time help you heal.

Dealing with emptiness and no purpose

There is an emptiness that comes with losing a loved one who we have been caring for. Usually, a carer is with the patient for over 40 or 50 hours a week or more if you sleep next to them at night. The carer's whole life begins to revolve around the needs and wants of the patient. You become each other's best friend, and you bicker with each other constantly. You are so in sync with each other that you start to know what they want before they know. You can almost know what they are thinking when they are silent or when you are away, you can sense that they are getting sicker or that they need you. You become inseparable and oh so dependent on each other.

Then, all of a sudden, one day, just like that, they are gone. Silent forever and just whoosh disappeared. You are left with nobody to care for and nothing to worry about or think about. But more than that, you are left without that person caring about you or worrying about you and looking out for you. There is a hole - a vast emptiness. In the blink of an eye, you are alone with no purpose, no meaning - and where there used to be so much to do and think about and plan and organise, there is a huge, empty void of nothingness.

Dealing with loss of attention from being with the patient

When we are a carer, we tend to get a lot of attention by hanging out with the patient. Especially if the patient has visually obvious signs of being ill, you will get treated like a VIP in the restaurants, on the road, pretty much everywhere. People will help you; they will get out of your way, they will hold the door, and they will give you preferential treatment in general. Without knowing it, you will get used to this special treatment. After the patient gets better or, God forbid, loses his/her life, this privilege will be lost, and you will become a regular person, one out of 8 billion. It is going to feel extremely strange not to be so entitled anymore; you will be brought back down to earth extremely fast.

You will probably be the centre of the patient's world, just like they are the centre of yours. This also will change abruptly. They may have tons of gratitude for what you did. They may even praise the hell out of you to everyone you know. They and the rest of the family won't know how to pay you back, but you will find yourself alone at the end of the day. They will get on with their own lives, and if you have not kept up with your people, your "tribe," and your friends, then I am afraid you will face lots of days of solitude and isolation. If we don't keep up with others and they aren't part of our journey in some way, it will be very hard to bridge the gap that has formed between us. You won't be able to relate to them, and they will find it extremely hard to relate to you if they haven't been through something similar or if you haven't shared any of your experiences or emotions with them along the way.

Dealing with a lack of gratitude and appreciation from others

On the other hand, you may face the opposite reaction. The family may not appreciate what you have done or your decisions. When we are going through the process of grief, there is a lot of denial and regret and loads of blaming and shaming. Unfortunately, if you end up a target of accusations from others, try to hold on to your anger and hurt. Everybody's minds are foggy right now, and they will have selective memories of the events that transpired. With time, they will see that everyone did their best in the moment with whatever information and experience they had under the circumstances. Like they say, in hindsight, everything is clear and makes sense, but we don't get to make decisions in hindsight. In the present, at the time of the decision, there are many variables and so many inputs that our decisions are influenced by. Therefore, we have to give it our best shot and then trust fate to do what is destined.

Dealing with having acquired knowledge and wanting to use it

Spending so much time in the hospital, dealing with doctors and nurses plus taking care of the patient at home with their medicines, their symptoms and reactions, makes us feel pretty much like semi-doctors ourselves. We become so attuned to every imbalance in the patient's moods, slight changes in behaviour which lend to a deep understanding of their health status.

We now have all the lingo down pact: CBC, WBC, kidney and liver profiles, blood pressure and glucose monitoring, breathing-related symptoms, differences between x-rays, MRI, CT scan with or without dye, PET scan, wound dressings, ultrasounds, bone scans, stents of all types, and the list goes on and on. We learn the difference between immunotherapy, chemotherapy, targeted therapy, variations of radiation (stereotactic or gamma knife), tumour-related vocabulary, and so much more. You learn that a lot of the chemotherapy meds sound like platinum (cisplatin), or they have the suffix -zumab or suffix -lutinib, and of course, there are bazillions out there.

We learn that diseases like diabetes can cause neuropathy in the legs, retinopathy in the eyes, cataracts, macular degeneration, retina detachment, etc. If we don't take care of the sugar, nerves stop feeling, eyes start blurring, infections turn into gangrene and amputations, and many people end up having to turn to dialysis to manually clean the kidney and remove toxins which affect the blood pressure. Or you could have wounds which have trouble healing and may heal with holes filled with infection after surgery, and the doctors come and re-open the wound, but this time without anaesthesia, and ask you to let them know as they are cutting your skin in front of you to let them know when it hurts. They only return the next day to continue where they left off. As the skin around all wounds becomes numb, they need to know when they reach the part that feels. Of course, the craziest of all is if you don't control your diabetes and your blood pressure decides to peak, that combination can cause a stroke! Or by luck, if you qualify for Whipple's Surgery to save yourself from pancreatic or bile duct cancer, then you will get what they call 'doctor-induced diabetes'. This requires you to learn a whole new method of using insulin to replace the fact that the patient doesn't have a pancreas and still needs to eat. In addition, the patient doesn't have enough digestive or pancreatic enzymes (suffix -ase ex amylase, lipase and protease), so you need to take Pancrelipase or Creons, preventing you from an upset stomach every time you eat.

Cystoscopies and prostate-related TURPS teach you that catheters can be taken home with you as long as you are able to handle changing the bags on your own. You learn that the chemo for bladder cancer is the BCG vaccination you got when you were a baby, and it left that weird mark on the side of your hip or arm. You learn that the chemo they use for serious cancers, Avastin, is used as an injection in your eye to reduce the inflammation in the back of your eye because you didn't get the right treatment when you got your cataract done. You learn that the pressure in your eye doesn't necessarily correlate with your blood pressure, but it does help to take the extra 5 mg of Norvasc or the generic name amlodipine to bring it down when it's very high. You learn that when you are wheezing, it's not always the case for a pulmonologist. Sometimes, it can be related to a gastric effect, and you will need to take nexium or the generic name omeprazole or rhyming thereof (ex, pantoprazole).

The wound -VAC is not a home vacuum but rather a wound vacuum and pulls out the blood and infection in a wound to help the wound heal better. But you also learn that once you step on the tube of the wound VAC by mistake and pop out the seal, you have a limited amount of time to get the dressing redone. If that is not possible, then nobody is going to do it for you, not even 911 or the emergency room nurses. You will have to take out the foam from a deep wound cavity, in this case, a cut from the chest to under the navel and deep enough for the doctor to put his hand inside. Then, you need to replace it with dry or wet gauze dressing instead so that the person doesn't get infected by the time you get an appointment with the wound department.

I think the most shocking realisation for me all across the board, whichever country we were in, every time you enter the hospital as a patient, they ask you what meds you are on and your history. What if you are passed out, I asked one of the nurses. She said we are trained to understand people's responses while they are not in their senses. How amazing that when we feel we are in a nonsensical state, they think they are wizards to understand something as important as which meds we take and our health history. Aren't those details a bit serious not to jump to conclusions rather than just looking up our history on the computer? Why can't we just have a device that updates our information, or why can't the information the patient gave in the last checkup be used?

At least that might be a close guess to what they are taking, rather than trying to guess their response when not in their senses.

Another issue that completely boggles my mind is that when a person gets administered chemo by the nurses, the nurses are not allowed to administer insulin to the patients in an out-patient chemo session. The crazy thing is that a lot of the patients are allergic to the stuff inside the chemo and are given strong antihistamines, which make them woozy and pass out. How are they supposed to check their own sugar and decide how many short-acting insulin units they need to inject themselves with to counteract the effect of the steroids in the chemo? (Steroids make the sugar level shoot up.)

CHAPTER 10

USES OF KNOWLEDGE:

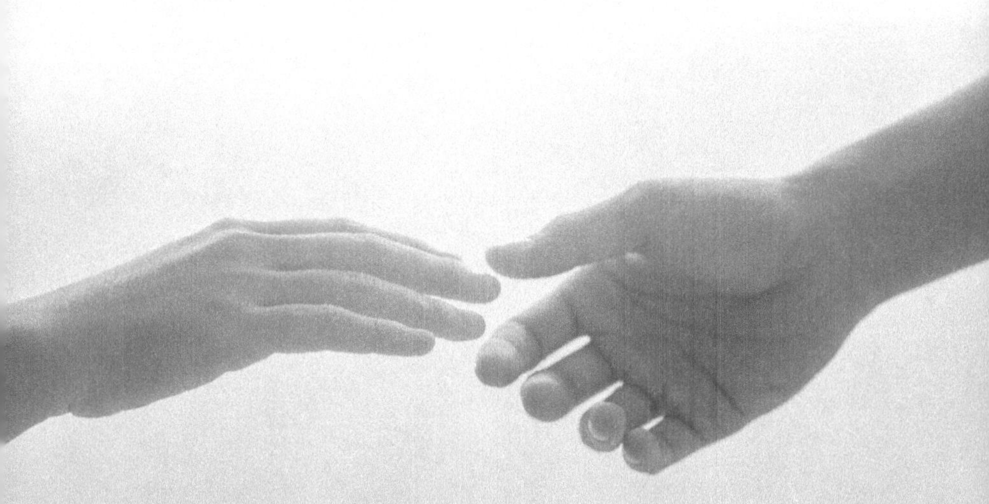

So the question is: what do we do with all this knowledge? We don't qualify as doctors, nor can we become nurses or consultants - for these, we don't have enough knowledge yet... after having dealt with so many hospitals around the world for bile duct cancer, bladder tumour, heart disease issues, lung cancers, diabetes-related retinopathy and surgery to remove boils, plus my own ripped Achilles tendon and surgery and collie's wrist with external implants, I felt like I could be a nurse. Clearly, it didn't qualify me anywhere near to being a nurse. Plus, after spending most of my life around people in hospitals, I don't feel like being around 'sad' situations anymore. It's like there was a limit to my empathy and patience, and I emptied that cup! Now, I just want to be happy and light about life.

I used to like being around people with issues to share their pain. I always felt bad for people suffering and always thought: I am so blessed, so I have to be there for people who aren't as blessed and lucky as I am. Even though it was a good thing, and people think I am great for doing what I did, I think it's not a good idea to give up your life fully the way I did. Of course, we must be there for our loved ones as we would love to have others be there for us. There are many situations where we cannot possibly take care of ourselves and need others to be there for us, there is no question about that.

I absolutely love my parents, and I do not regret being there for them at all, but I think there has to be a way where it's not just one person who loses their life fully taking care of the parents. They are everyone's parents, and the duty is everyone's, and it should be shared. No one's life should come to a standstill while others are living their lives to show up only in emergencies and when they have time. No one can compare their input with yours unless they are sharing the time of caregiver duties with you equally. So if they haven't, let them know - give them a chance to do it. Then, if they don't, they can't compare their experience with yours. One can never know what it feels like until one has done it in the same capacity.

After the initial few years of grieving, I went through a deep, dark phase. In this phase, all I wanted was to end my life, but clearly, this isn't very easy to do. Plus, my religion and spiritual self would never allow this. After ten days of the darkest period of my life and praying as hard as I could with tons and tons of gratitude, I started bouncing upwards from rock bottom. All of a sudden, I realised I had this new energy and freedom to do whatever I wanted, and all I wanted to do was everything I could.

Not only did I lose my relatives and had all this grief to deal with, but now I also had lost my youth and had that to grieve about. When a parent or loved one gets diagnosed with a life-threatening disease, your first thought is not about, "Oh my God, what about me?" The intensity of the situation makes your body freeze, and the severity of the situation causes you to go into fight or flight mode. Your brain freezes, and your heart explodes with pain, love, and fear, all at once, with sympathy for the patient. You wonder:

1) How will they take the news?

2) How will they deal with the fact that they may not be here

indefinitely? (We tend to think we are immortal when we are healthy.)

3) How will they take the physical, mental and emotional pains involved in the journey of getting treated and having to deal with all the different experiences yet to come?

4) How much will they suffer through surgeries, procedures, treatments, etc?

5) How long do they have? (The biggest question of them all, which doesn't have an answer until it actually happens.)

6) How do we talk about difficult issues like mortality, leaving loved ones, wills and other big decisions?

7) How will they deal with the spiritual and/or religious aspects of the journey yet to come?

8) Will the patient be able to endure the pain and suffering yet to come?

9) Will you be able to be there for them and how much?

10) Will you be able to be their strength in their tough times and not fall apart?

11) Will you be able to hold back your tears in front of them while your heart is paining incessantly for them while knowing the inevitable is always around the corner?

12) How much love can I give them before…?

Every day, every emergency, every skipped breath, every gasp while sleeping, every fall, every time they pass out, every surgery… the ominous feeling is felt beneath the hope the doctors provide. As much as the statistics appease our logical side, our emotional side cries, "But what if…?" Nobody voices it, yet everyone feels it. It is always the elephant in the room. A diagnosis of cancer, rare diseases, stroke, leukaemia and all other scary, life-threatening diseases just come and hit you in the gut: it literally feels like a death sentence. As much as we and the doctors like to sugar-coat it for the patient and ourselves, superficially discussing statistics of survival and beautiful remissions and cures, the underlying wrench keeps twisting everyone inside as the ominous option of death hovers constantly. Yet, no one has the guts to face it or even think in that direction.

Why are we so scared of death and of talking about it? The only thing we know when we are born is that we are going to die. There is no other guarantee in life. Whether one is religious or not, once we are born, the only thing God promises us is that we are going to die one day. Nothing in between is a right or a given, anything can happen in between, no one has a clue. Yet we ignore the death part as if this life is all that matters, and we live like we are never going to die. Yet we see and hear in the news all the time that people of all ages are losing their lives to diseases, wars, and accidents regardless of age limits. Children die before their parents, parents die when children are young, there is no set sequence to predict.

I can go through as much loss and grief as possible, but it will never make me an expert on grief. Everyone's grief and everyone's way of dealing with it is personal and unique - we cannot and should not compare. Not only that, but my own grief changed depending on my relationship with each person who passed. Every relationship of mine that I lost to death had a completely different impact on my life and my emotions. The way a person passes also has a special impact on those of us who are left behind. My mother's illness gave us a warning for 2 and a half years to spoil her and make amends, but for her, there was a lot of suffering. My dad, on the other hand, left us in limbo, disappearing in a flash in his sleep. No warning, no preparation, no time to make amends or say goodbye, but for him, it was the easiest and best way to leave us without suffering. Complete, polar opposite ways of departure from this world.

Why don't we think of birth as an illness? Isn't it so when we think about it? As soon as we are born, we die a little and get a day closer to death, whatever day that may be. Why do we wait till someone gets sick to be nice to them and forgive them? Why do we wait for those moments to pack all our love and care in? Why do we let our ego control our lives when things are 'normal'? Why is it so easy to let go when someone is dying, yet impossible to soften when everyone is healthy and strong? If only we could mend our relationships before life makes us succumb, we would not have regrets, allowing us to carry our loved ones to their inevitable destination with peace and calm.

What now?

Reaching here will be one of the toughest journeys you will have crossed in your life: financially, emotionally, mentally and physically. These situations are firsts for most people, so don't be hard on yourself if you don't know how to handle them. It's imperative that you start to focus on healing from the traumas you have experienced. It may be something everyone goes through, but it's still a trauma.

First and foremost, you should try to talk to people who can relate to your situation. Knowing that other people have gone through the same feelings and confusion that you are going through will already make you feel better. Like they say, 'misery loves company'. In a sense, you will feel a semblance of being 'normal' once you know you are not alone in feeling the way you do. Secondly, please don't shy away from getting therapy to help you learn how to deal with it. Therapists will listen to you and guide you. They may not resolve all your issues, but they will provide you with a map of how you should proceed. Lastly, hold on to your faith and/or spiritual rituals and traditions. Therapy and friends can only lead you to part of the path, the rest is only figured out by holding the guiding hand of the One above.

In your times of solitude and reflection, when anxiety takes over your body and mind, He is the only one who can give you relief and provide peace in your heart. His presence looms over you as consistently as you breathe, and His love envelopes you constantly, even when you forget He is there. His promise to be there for you is the most unconditional and trustworthy promise to bet on in your life. Take advantage of the peace and nurturing He has offered you, and you will feel calm within and will not get overpowered by any sort of negativity whatsoever. He is the most consistent friend and love you will ever have, reach out to Him - He is waiting for you.

Experiencing the loss of a parent and spending days or years at the hospital, seeing them degenerate in front of your eyes changes you. It changes the core of your personality, it changes the way you think and it inevitably changes the way you look at the world and the people around you. You might find that your friends are nice, but they aren't on the same wavelength as you. You may not connect with them the way you used to anymore. Getting back to 'real life' will be greatly impacted. You might even have a change of heart and reconsider your purpose in life. Perhaps you will change jobs or roles in life; anything can happen since now you are a different person than when you started this journey. It's time to get to know yourself again!

About The Author

I am a Canadian citizen, born in Kinshasa, Democratic Republic of Congo. My lineage can be traced to Gujarat, India, yet some of my relatives live in Karachi, Pakistan. I went to an American School, a Canadian University for my undergrad and then to an English University for my MEd., in Dubai, UAE, which is where I currently live. I speak English, French, Lingala, Urdu and Gujarati, and I understand bits of Arabic and Swahili.

Having lived in many different cities around the world and having travelled widely, I feel like a global citizen connected to everyone everywhere. My mission in life is to provide support to as many people as I can by creating support groups and communities for carers to come together all across the world. Let's care for carers too!

About The Book

God forbid when someone in the family gets diagnosed with a chronic or fatal illness, the entire family comes together for a few days. The entire load of the patient's care will go on one of the family members who will spend the most time, money, energy and/or emotions in the process while becoming the caregiver. Everyone will focus on caring for the patient while the care for the carer is neglected. Why don't we try caring for the carer for a change?

This book shares some ideas on how a carer can care for the patient in addition to caring for themselves in the process. This book is a must-read for everyone who has someone suffering in the family with a chronic illness. Allow me tell you that you are not alone while reading my experiences through this book. Let's come together and share our journeys.